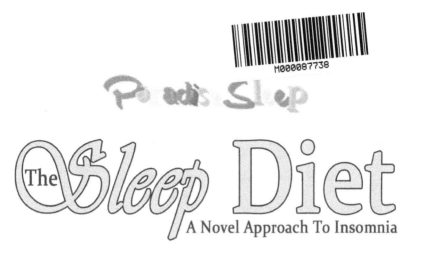

Paradis Sleep

The Sleep Diet
A Novel Approach To Insomnia

José Colón M.D., MPH

Halo ●●●●
Publishing International

ISBN: 978-1-61244-230-3
Library of Congress Control Number: 2013918804

Printed in the United States of America

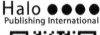

Published by Halo Publishing International
AP# 726
P.O Box 60326
Houston, Texas 77205
Toll Free 1-877-705-9647
Website: www.halopublishing.com
E-mail: contact@halopublishing.com

I dedicate this book to my wife, Krystal
and to my kids, Manuel and Jada—Love.

Table of Contents

Foreword

Insomnia is a very difficult process to go through. There are physical and emotional pains that accompany it. My compassion goes to everyone who has suffered from sleeplessness and/or sleepiness.

I have seen the face of distress and heard the plea for sleep. One would never wish insomnia on anyone, yet one wishes the people around them could understand the agony.

At times we self-medicate and though we may feel occasional relief, the beast of insomnia with its racing thoughts still seems to catch up to us. Other times we go to our doctor for help. When medicine helps, we feel great. But it doesn't always work out that way.

Many books define insomnia, but no definition explains a feeling. I know what it is like wanting to sleep with a mind racing. This was before my exposure to behavioral sleep medicine. In my desire to reach out and help, I have written this book.

Who has time to read about the insomnia we loathe? By now, you have already looked online and read about sleep tips. If you've already read a sleep book, it may have put you to sleep in the daytime, yet failed to do so in the night when you desire your mind to rest. My friends, this is why I took a "novel" approach to insomnia.

Imagination is more important than knowledge. Logic will get you from A to B. Your imagination will take you everywhere.
—Albert Einstein

If you have insomnia, I hope my book benefits you. *Note: it is not a traditional instructional book. I say this because this does not replace professional care.*

I made an early observation about my sleep patients. They are sleepy! Even the most interested and engaged person can eventually drift into a drowsy state with slow roving eye movements. If this book seems fragmented, it is by design. Sleepy people may need to take regular mental breaks. My method is to provide mental breaks between chapters to stay focused, as well as to provide pearls at the end of each chapter. And anyone can subscribe to receive *Paradise Sleep Pearls* on www.ParadiseSleep.com.

If you do not have insomnia, I wish three things. One, my book entertains you. Two, you understand and can have compassion for friends or loved ones that do. Three, you never develop insomnia based on the lessons learned in this book.

I'm Dr. Jose Colon. Sleep medicine is my passion. Improving family health through sleep science education is my mission.

Paradise Sleep Pearls: The number of zolpidem-related ER visits is rising according to a 2013 report by The Substance Abuse and Mental Health Services Administration. Even more alarming, a potential long-term side effect of sleeping pills is increased mortality.

We can't solve problems by using the same kind of thinking we used when we created them.
—Albert Einstein

1. Zolpidem-related ER Visits Rise Sharply. sleepreviewmag.com 2013
2. Kripke, DF. 2007. Hypnotics versus the alternatives. Psychiatric Investigations 4:57-60
3. Kripke, DF. Et al. 2002 Mortality associated with sleep duration and insomnia. Archives of General Psychiatry, 59:131-36

Success and Accomplishment

"Patience, Valium and a mimosa," Mellissa hears when her friend Jez answers Mellissa's call.

"What?" Mellissa says back. "How about a simple 'hello' or maybe a 'good morning'?"

Jez laughs. "I'm a nurse who works both days and nights, and last night was a long night. On my way out, I was asked if I needed anything and I responded, 'patience, Valium and a mimosa.' I kind of liked the ring of it."

"Sorry to hear you had a long night, Jez." Mellissa knows sometimes Jez needs to let off some steam after a night shift at the hospital. "I hope you're able to get some sleep. I know that's been tough with your days and nights mixed up."

"I'm fine. It was a long night, but I love what I do. Funny though, I've been sleeping great the last month ever since I was given Valium."

"You don't really mix it with mimosas, do you?"

"No way! It was just the first thing that came to my mind as I looked out the window and saw people coming into the hospital this morning with orange juice. What about you? How have you been?"

"You know, it's been a tough time with my worries about getting the promotion, but I got it," Mellissa says. "I'm senior marketing partner now!"

"That is awesome, Mellissa! Success and accomplishment is what you are all about. I can't think of any obstacle you have come across that you haven't persevered through. I know you have lost sleep over the promotion—I've seen your Facebook posts! Hey, why don't you ask your doctor about a sleep med?"

"Thanks for the encouragement. You're a good friend and I actually have my yearly physical coming up tomorrow. But…I don't think I need a sleep med. I've tried melatonin already. My sister Dedee insists she needs to take it every night to relax, but it hasn't worked for me. It's the worrying about my position in the company that has kept me up just about every night for the past year since our boss announced he was going to retire. Now that's settled, I figure I can finally sleep."

"I know you are better at what you do than your male colleague, what is his name? Bud?"

"Barry. He has more seniority, but less creativity. He also whines a lot about the travel. What else would you expect when you work in the resort and vacation industry? I'm actually heading out again later this week. It will be our first quarterly meeting with me running the show. I really have lost so much sleep over this promotion."

"Well, now you have your promotion. Now you can finally just relax."

"I can't wait to get some sleep tonight. I'm even going to go to bed early. I was calling to see if you wanted to get together tomorrow night. Rick will be at the fire station. Maybe we could get a drink and celebrate."

"Sorry, but no can do. I'm scheduled to work the next two nights. Thanks for asking. Now, I need to go home, take my Valium and get some shut-eye. I'm actually looking forward to working with this new doctor, a woman. It will be nice to have another female around and not hear 'girls' every time the doctor needs something."

"How long do you plan to work those overnight shifts?" Mellissa asks.

"I don't know. John and I were talking about it. We were thinking about starting a family."

"Oh, that's great! Have you guys been trying already?"

"No," says Jez. "I just stopped my birth control last month. Your sister told me all you have to do is just stop trying to prevent it. What about you? You guys have been talking about a family for some time now."

Mellissa looks down, her head and shoulders fall. She exhales. "Maybe we can get together next week after my quarterly meeting."

Paradise Sleep Pearls: Insomnia is the most common sleep complaint in the industrialized world—about 40% of the population and about 70% never discuss this with their doctor. So what is the pearl? You are not alone!

1. Sateia MJ, Doghramji K, Hauri PJ, Morin CM. Evaluation of chronic insomnia. An American Academy of Sleep Medicine review. SLEEP 2000; 23(2):243-308.
2. Ancoli-Israel S, Roth T. Characteristics of insomnia in the United States: results of the 1991 National Sleep Foundation Survey. SLEEP 1999; 22(suppl 2):S347-S353.

Why Can't I Relax?

Why can't I relax? Why can't I relax? Why can't I relax? Mellissa pleads to herself, wide-eyed as she lies bundled in bed watching her husband Rick sleep with envy. She forces her eyelids shut, inviting the darkness. *Sleeping requires doing absolutely nothing. Nothing! Why can't I do nothing? Insomnia is a bitch!*

After a few breaths, the darkness of her closed eyes becomes a distant memory as her eyes pop open again.

She swiftly rolls over facing her husband. She tugs at the sheets, wrapping herself snugly. As she closes her eyes once more, Rick snores loudly and her eyes fly open again. She rolls onto her back. The popcorn-white ceiling stares back at her. There is a hint of yellow light coming from the bathroom. She closes her eyes again. Rick snores again, right on cue.

Wide-eyed once again, Mellissa lies back down and stares through the sheer curtains over the window above her bed at the yellow street lamp and the white moon. She fans the sheets and comforter a couple of times and then rolls onto her side. Now facing her night table again, Mellissa suddenly notices the glowing green numbers on her clock: *2:00 am!* She rolls her eyes. She calculates she has been in bed for three hours.

She rolls back to her other side to face Rick. Though he appears to be snoring peacefully, the noise is making it impossible for her to sleep. Mellissa debates whether to pinch the snore from his nose. She brings her other hand's index finger to her mouth, prepared to shush him once he awakens from the nose pinch. She knows he won't see the humor in this at 2 am. Instead, she gently pulsates his shoulder, urging, "You're snoring on your back again. Roll over!"

"Huh?" replies her husband in sleep drunkenness. He hardly ever remembers these interactions the next morning. "I already told you, I want steak for dinner." He then obediently rolls to his side and the snoring ceases.

He's probably dreaming of one of his steaks he posts on Facebook. How am I supposed to get to sleep when he's snoring and talking in his sleep? In the sudden quiet, Mellissa debates whether or not to stay in bed, knowing it's only a matter of time before the snoring starts up again. She kicks off the sheets and gets out of bed. She snags her pillow and her phone with the other hand as she makes her routine migration to the living room couch.

As she passes down the hall, she is drawn to the clock. "2:20 am," she sighs. At the end of the hallway is a full-length mirror. She stops and stares at her reflection up close. Even in the near-complete darkness, she can see the darker areas under her eyes. The longer she stares at them, the darker they become and when they seem as dark as her long black hair, she breaks eye contact with the mirror and continues her nightly trek.

Arriving at the couch, Mellissa throws down her pillow and plops down next to it. She stretches her legs out in front of her and wiggles her toes. She covers herself with a fuzzy red throw blanket draped over the back of the couch, kicking aside the insomnia self-help book she had left on the couch the prior evening. The book falls to the floor, opening to the first chapter revealing the bookmark in the spine. *If only sleep would come to me just by opening the book.*

Mellissa closes her eyes desperate to find rest. She feels the breeze from the ceiling fan brush her nose, triggering her eyes to open. Her eyelids close again. Hearing the soft clang of the fan's chain banging against the body of the fan, her eyes open once again, seemingly of their own accord. Her attention suddenly fixates on the sway of the chain. Her eyes follow it back and forth until they close again.

She focuses on the rhythm of the fan's swivel in concert with the clang of the chain and the breeze on her nose. Once again, her eyes pop open staring at the revolving fan blades. She reaches to the floor to pick up the insomnia book, thinking it might actually be good to read it now—since it seems to bore her to sleep during the day. The thought of reading when she is tired is too much and instead she tucks it under her pillow, hoping its contents will enter her brain through osmosis.

Mellissa suddenly sits up on the couch and picks the laptop up from the coffee table. Placing it on her lap, she presses the power button and waits for it to boot up. Leaning her head back and resting it against the back of the couch. The chiming of her computer announces she is logged on and goes to Facebook. She longs to see the green dot next to the name of one of her friends indicating someone else is up and available to chat. Mellissa's sister used to be up frequently at this time because her young daughter would keep her up. Since Dedee had another baby six months ago, she is too busy at night to get online.

Mellissa clicks in the status update box at the top of the page. 2:40 am and I'm awake again! Another sleepless night in Nashville: she posts. *Besides, if I am up, someone else should be. And misery loves company. In the middle of the night with Rick snoring, online company is better than the silence of the living room or the snoring in the bedroom.* Tonight the silence in her living room apparently has extended to a silence online as well.

Mellissa looks around, eyes stopping at the TV. She reaches for the remote, but she can't reach it and doesn't feel like getting up. She lunges one last time, this time hearing her polished fingernail hitting the remote and pushing it farther away. She sits back on the sofa in defeat and decides to scroll through her unviewed Facebook notifications instead.

Mellissa posted earlier that day she was going to ask about planning a pregnancy at her annual physical tomorrow—well, today now. Only Dedee knows they have actually been trying to conceive for a few years. Mellissa sees Rick's sister-in-law had responded: You don't plan on having a baby. You just stop trying to prevent it.

Her husband, Rick's brother, also had a comment: If you plan it right, you can have three kids in diapers at the same time.

That's just not funny. Mellissa exits out of her notifications.

Mellissa looks at her clock again. "Ugh! It's 2:50 am," she whispers. Reluctantly she gets up to grab the remote from the coffee table. She turns on the TV, which was apparently on MTV when it was last on. She hopes for a little music to put her to sleep but sees instead the reality show *16 and Pregnant* is on.

She flicks the TV off just as fast as she turned it on.

Mellissa's head lowers and she moves her elbows to her knees, resting her face on all ten fingertips. *All you have to do is close your eyes and go to sleep. Stop using birth control and get pregnant. Now I have a doctor's appointment tomorrow, but I'm going to be exhausted. I'm going to be too tired to understand anything he says and I will never get pregnant.* Mellissa's mind races and she can't stop it.

"I need a cigarette!" She says aloud, getting up and walking to the front porch.

Rick doesn't like the smell of cigarettes and it hurts when he refers to it as a "stench" and asks her why she can't quit altogether. She doesn't want to deal with any further negativity about something she doesn't feel like she has control over so she sneaks outside to enjoy her nightly cigarette. *It's just one, after all.* She passes by the laundry room and grabs her pajama sweats from the dryer. She slips on the bottoms over her work out shorts before making her way to the porch and lighting up.

I wish I never posted we are trying to have kids. Last thing I need are jokes and unsolicited advice. Mellissa is 29. Dedee is 26 and has a three-year-old and a six-month-old.

Mellissa huffs her cigarette, the orange-red end pulsating in intensity with her inhalations. She used to enjoy this more but smoking has turned into a chore, done in a rush to finish before Rick catches her smoking. She rubs the lit end out on the damp outdoor rail and brings it inside to the bathroom. The evidence flushes down the toilet, but she can still smell the smoke. Tucking her long, straight hair behind her ears, Mellissa uses lavender soap and warm water to wash her face and hands. *Lavender soap makes everyone sleep except for me.*

Suddenly, she feels her heart fall to the pit of her stomach as panic sets in. *He's going to leave me if I'm unable to give him a baby.* She feels her heart rattle and stares at her own ashen face. After a few moments, she realizes the water is still pouring from the faucet and quickly turns it off. She dries her face on the bathroom towel and dries her hands off on her sweatshirt as she walks to the bedroom.

Mellissa opens the bedroom door and hears snoring. She exhales through her nose and shakes her head, shutting the door, turning back around and making her trek to the quiet couch. She avoids the hall mirror this time, but can't avoid eyeing the living room clock as she plops back down on the couch.

Lying back down, she feels something hard under the pillow. She reaches underneath, pulling the insomnia book out, placed there for good luck earlier. She tosses it back to the ground. Twisting her body toward the back of the couch, she hears the thud of the book hitting the floor.

Why can't I relax? Why can't I relax? Why can't I relax? Mellissa obsesses as she clenches her eyes tight. *I just have to try harder. Insomnia is a bitch!*

Paradise Sleep Pearls: Neurological research suggests brain "hyperarousal" is associated with insomnia. The way I like to explain this is by comparing "brain rhythms" with heart rates. Just as we have a heart rate, we also have brain rhythms that influence brain arousal. Another way to view the term "brain arousal" is by our level of alertness. As we rest, our heart rate generally slows as does our brain rhythms. Emotions such as fear, agitation and anxiety cause your heart rate to speed up. Those same emotions increase the level of our brain arousal.

Sleep in America; 1995. Princeton, NJ: The Gallup Organization, 1995.

What a Girl Needs

"Mel Honey, you fell asleep on the couch again. And your alarm woke me up, again." Mellissa hears Rick saying to her.

"Ugh!" says Mellissa, bolting upright and grabbing her phone, realizing from its display not only had she fallen asleep on the couch, but also slept through the phone alarm clock. Using two alarms helps to keep her from continuing to hit the snooze. "Who would be able to sleep through your snoring? You could've woken the dead last night. I thought I told you to get that checked out?"

Mellissa jumps up from the couch, upset about getting a late start to her day. She scurries to the coffeemaker but ends up feeling as if she is walking underwater. After loading the coffeemaker she leans over the counter, resting her head on her hands to take the stress off her neck as she waits for the coffee to percolate.

"I told you I don't snore," Rick says. "And even if I did, I can't wear that Darth Vader mask anyway. You know I'm claustrophobic."

"You mean you don't *hear* yourself snoring!" Mellissa snaps. She pours her first cup of coffee, thinking about the invisible band of throbbing pressure around her head. "And you don't hear yourself talking in your sleep, either. I do and it keeps me awake. I'm just going to move my stuff to the couch and sleep there from now on. Good luck trying to conceive a child when we're sleeping in different rooms."

"Mel Honey, don't go there. I'm not pressuring you about having kids," Rick eases.

"Your mother is. Your father is. Your brother is...and even your sister-in-law is," Mellissa replies.

Mellissa's husband moves towards her gently and takes her chin in his hand. He looks her in the eye and with a light-hearted facial expression. He speaks calmly. "They aren't me, baby. And they're not pressuring. We just come from a big family and we love kids. People talk about what they love. Take it with a grain of salt." He smiles at her, rubbing her back with his other hand.

Gradually Rick's conciliatory body language transfers to Mellissa. As the furrows of her forehead relax so does the tension around her ears and neck.

"I know, I know," Mellissa says, stepping toward him. She puts her arms around him, laying her head on his left shoulder and with a deep breath, closes her eyes.

"How's your nook, babe? Is that what you needed?" He whispers in her ear.

"I love my nook," she says. "It's always exactly what I need. But you know you'll have to share it one day if we have a little girl."

"Nah. I only make boys," he teases.

"OK, macho man." Mellissa laughs.

"Sorry you couldn't sleep last night." Rick pats her back, then pauses and looks at her curiously. "What happened to your insomnia book? Isn't it the second one you've tried?"

"It's hopeless." Mellissa lifts her head and releases from his embrace. She walks to the couch and picks up the book. "The first one talked about natural herbs and remedies. I already tried them all before I even went through the entire book. This new one is just boring. And it's too long. They should understand that people with insomnia are too tired to sit down and read."

"Then shouldn't it help to put you to sleep?"

Mellissa exhales and shakes her head. "If only it were that easy. I wish you understood." She turns and starts to head to the bedroom to get ready.

"I love you, Mel Honey. I'm trying to understand," Rick says as he follows her.

At the doorway to the hallway, Mellissa stops and turns around. She looks at the book lying forlornly on the ground by the couch and then looks back at him. "You have no idea what it feels like to be exhausted to the point where your mind feels foggy. And what it's like to know all you have to do is close your eyes but somehow when you close your eyes, your mind just won't shut down: work; infertility; family; gossip. All you want to do is get up and…and…" Mellissa pauses to keep herself from adding about the cigarette. "And find somebody to talk to," she goes on. "But who else is up in the middle of the night? No-body. So you keep trying. You open your eyes and look around to stop the racing thoughts, but your eyelids are heavy and the longer you keep them open, the more the fog builds."

"Sounds like a Catch-22 of misery." Rick approaches her again and grabs her hand. "I'm sorry. If I could give you my sleep, I would. Why don't you ask your doctor about it today?"

"Yeah, Jez was given Valium and she claims she has been sleeping great this past month." Mellissa exhales and shakes her head again. "But I'm a mess. I have a hard enough time understanding his medical mumbo jumbo and I'm exhausted on top of it. I already have to ask him about infertility. I don't know if I'll have time to ask him about both that and the insom-nia. He was so rushed when I saw him last year for my annual physical."

"Well, try to make sure he makes time." Rick pats her hand. "Jez is a crazy girl. But she has been a really good friend to you."

"Yeah, since high school, you know? We used to stay up all night talking about life and our futures. Up all night willingly if you can imagine that."

"Oh! I've been meaning to ask you, why don't we have a New Year's party at our place?"

Mellissa's head pops back. "Oh, please no. If I have the usual bad night of sleep…I just told you I'm exhausted." Mellis-sa gets nervous at the thought. Her sleep is so unpredictable.

She never knows if she will get a normal eight hours or if her mind won't slow down and cause her to be up all night. "I would never be able to stay up that late. I love the kids but when they are up late, they get hyperactive. Then all the men tell the kids to get their mother. I end up stuck with the girls and they have all these kids with energy crawling out of their skin. They either climb on me or keep saying, 'Look at me! Look at me!' I can't deal with that at our place. It's not as if I can just leave our house and sleep somewhere else." Mellissa feels her stomach move as she explains.

"I just thought it would be fun to hang out with all our friends."

"I know but not at night. I'm sorry. I thought I would sleep better after my promotion. If it didn't happen last night, after feeling so relieved, I don't think it will happen any night. I think I've forgotten how to sleep."

Rick doesn't say a word. He just looks at her with interest and concern.

"Thanks for listening to me," she says. They hug again. "You know what I really need?"

"Morning love?" replies Rick, grabbing hold of her hands and gently tugging her towards the bedroom.

"No! I need to go shopping. I need to get some new gym clothes."

"Oh…I was going to invite you to shower with me to conserve water. And after the shower…oh wait. You're going to the doctor today so you can't."

"No. It's not that type of checkup. It's just my yearly physical—but I need to address trying to get pregnant."

"So you can have some morning love!" A huge grin spreads across Rick's face. "What did you just say you were going to ask about again? Hmm? Hmm?" He again pulls her toward the bedroom. "You're already halfway there since you don't have any pajamas on. Plus it will make you feel better."

"You know I don't ever sleep with pajamas and you can't expect me to be in the mood after the night I had." Mellissa releases Rick's hands.

"I'm sorry. I just feel that way sometimes first thing in the morning." Rick shrugs his shoulders and grins.

Mellissa shakes her head and turns away. *Why does every man want to have sex at any point in the day, especially in the morning?* She restarts her trek to the bedroom, hoping for a little privacy, trying to ignore Rick adjusting himself. When she looks back, Rick is still tailing her.

"Why haven't you been sleeping with your pajama sweats lately?" Rick tries to restart the conversation.

"I like to be able to get up and run, but lately my running skirts and shorts have zippers that snag the throw blanket on the couch. And in the bed the material makes me slip around too much." Mellissa continues walking to the bedroom. "I need to get ready. I'm running late for my appointment."

Rick stops following her. "Are you going to get any blood-work done today?"

"Stop it!" Mellissa turns around wide-eyed and looks at Rick. "You know I can pass out just with the thought of having bloodwork done. I'm not a nurse like Jez."

"Sorry. Don't know how you ever made it through that bee tattoo on your foot."

"That's different. I love honeybees. And the blend of cosmos and pear martinis before helped."

"I love you," Rick says as he walks back to the coffee machine. "I'll make you an extra cup of your elixir of life. You know it's going to be a while before I make you coffee again, since you're going out of town."

"I guess it will be a little while 'till I see you again."

"I plan to catch up on my saltwater aquarium business while you're gone. It's really taking off. I have a couple of maintenance jobs to do tomorrow. I love the colors of the aquariums. I also love the early work hours, since I usually have to complete my job before each business opens for the day."

"You've always been an early bird," Mellissa replies.

"And you used to be a night owl. You think that's why you have problems sleeping at night?"

"I don't know, maybe. After my father passed away, I would stay up late until my mom came home from working at the restaurant to watch TV with me, 'till I fell asleep."

Mellissa finally turns on the shower then scurries to get her clothes together as she waits for the water to get hot. She takes out some gym clothes to go running after her appointment. She looks at her gym clothes and thinks to herself, *I love you too, Lululemon. I know you understand me.*

As Mellissa gets ready, she goes to her bathroom to take her ritual monthly pregnancy test—mostly because she has pregnancy on her mind, but also because her menstrual cycle has never been regular. Mellissa sets the test down on the counter. The steam on the bathroom window indicates the water is hot and she proceeds to the shower. In a mad dash, she leaves before going back and seeing the result, something she commonly does.

Paradise Sleep Pearls: Insomnia can have negative daytime issues as well. These may include memory difficulties, concentration problems, mood problems, poor work performance, problems in relationships, daytime drowsiness and headaches.

Sleep in America; 1995. Princeton, NJ: The Gallup Organization, 1995

I'm Not Depressed

Mellissa sits in the exam room wearing only a paper gown and shivering. Her feet are cold. She updates her Facebook status: I need a runner's high. Mellissa craves a good run through Centennial Park around the ponds and flowers. She likes how the park has many different paths, rather than being like a maze with dead ends, it is labyrinth like, always leading back to the middle.

Mellissa shivers on the cold exam table. The crinkling of exam paper matches the sound of her stomach rumbles. *Why do they even schedule 9 am appointments when you don't get seen 'till after 10 am?* "So annoying," she says aloud. There's a knock at the door.

"I'm sorry, Mellissa," says the doctor. "Busy. There just isn't enough hours in the day. And then people show up late, they show up on time, they show up early…sometimes even on the wrong day, but always want to be seen at the same time."

Is this an excuse? Mellissa responds, "I understand." She feels the throbbing band around her head returning due to the unlucky combination of poor sleep and not eating at her normal time.

"Your blood pressure is good," says her doctor, looking at the chart. "Let's do your physical." He examines her heart with a cold stethoscope, listens to her breathing and checks her neck. "No swollen lymph nodes." He then pulls out a thin plastic instrument resembling the plastic of a price tag and examines the bottom of her feet with it.

"That always tickles. Why exactly do you do that?"

"Elderly people can lose feeling in their feet. Happens more commonly with diabetes," her doctor replies in a monotone manner.

I'm not elderly and I don't have diabetes, but who am I to question the doctor in his white coat? Great the eye-looker-thinger. That light is like gasoline on the fire of my headaches. "I have contacts in," says Mellissa. Her intention is for him to realize she goes to an eye doctor so he doesn't need to shine the blinding light in her eyes.

"Can you see through your contacts?" the doctor asks.

"Well, yes."

"Then so can I," he replies.

Mellissa feels dumb and can't even muster the energy to express the headache. She feels awkward when her doctor is suddenly eye-to-eye, almost nose to nose, with exception of the bright light slowly burning a hole in her eye and blinding her. A mental image of a kid holding a magnifying glass on the concrete trying to burn ants appears, only the light ends up deflecting off the ants and into the back of her eye. This makes her already tense neck get tighter and the migraine throb harder. A lingering scent of Listerine from his breath adds an ice pick like feature to her headache.

"Anything going on?" asks her doctor as he begins to blind her other eye.

"I can't get pregnant," says Mellissa.

"Have you been trying?"

Mellissa finds this an awkward question.

"Yes, probably too much," Mellissa replies, although she is sure her husband would disagree.

"Well, maybe you should see a fertility specialist. I have a good friend in mind. I think he could get you pregnant."

Awkward! Did you not hear what you just said? She replies, "OK."

"Good. I will have the girls up front give you a referral. He can get you pregnant. He actually got two of the girls in our office pregnant."

"TMI," Mellissa says.

"You have TMJ too?" asks her doctor.

"No. I'm sorry. I don't know what I was saying." Mellissa feels heat rising to her checks.

"OK. No jaw pain," says her doctor. "No other complaints. Good. We are done. Girls up front will take care of you."

"Doc, I can't sleep at night."

"You could be depressed. We should have you see a psychiatrist."

"I don't feel depressed. I just have problems sleeping. I've tried everything: Melatonin, over the counter sleep aids, red wine, cherry juice, chamomile tea—and many different herbals."

"Have you tried Melatonin?" he asks.

"Excuse me? Yes. I just told you."

"Well, we should also have you see a psychiatrist to find out why you are depressed."

"But I don't feel depressed!" Mellissa snaps. After a short pause, she brings the palm of her hands up in attempt to calm herself. "I want to be respectful of people with depression. My sister has suffered through depression. But I'm telling you, I don't feel depressed. I just can't sleep."

"Depression is very commonly genetic. Do you feel fatigued in the day?"

"Yes, but really it's when I don't sleep."

"Do you spend a lot of time in bed?" asks her doctor. "Other than trying to get pregnant?"

"Well, yeah. I guess. I mean it takes me a lot of time to get to sleep so I go to bed early. And on weekends, I try to sleep in as late as I can since I didn't sleep well all week. But I still just can't sleep."

"Do you have insomnia?"

Mellissa stares at him with her mouth open. *I just told him that I cannot sleep and then he asked me if I have insomnia.* Her doctor barely meets her eyes and wears the same facial expression from the moment he entered the room. Mellissa is speechless.

"Look, I have other patients," says her doctor, eyeing his watch. "A psychiatrist can help you understand why you are sad. Many women your age go through depression. Especially when they can't conceive. How old are you again?"

Mellissa is flabbergasted. "I'm…I'm 29."

"That's right, you are about to turn 30," says her doctor. "Haven't you been on an antidepressant before? Do you have stress in your life?"

"Hasn't everyone been on an antidepressant before at one time in their life?" Mellissa shrugs her shoulders with her palms up. "Is it common to get depressed when you turn 30? Do all your patients go through this?"

"I don't typically ask," the doctor replies, making his way toward the door. "Look, I have to go see other patients. I will have your psychiatry and fertility referrals up at the front. They can help find out what is wrong with you and maybe the two of them together can get you pregnant."

Mellissa leans forward, tearing the paper garment as the doctor attempts to scurry out the door. "I have a friend who couldn't sleep and her doctor gave her Valium. Now she is sleeping well. Do you think you can provide that for me? Or is there a doctor that specializes in sleep?"

Her doctor stops, removes his hand from the door handle without closing the door and turns back around. He exhales and frowns. *That's the first change in his expression she has seen today—or maybe even in a few years.*

"You don't need a sleep study since you don't snore."

He didn't even ask me if I snore. She remembers about her husband's snoring and wants to ask further, but doesn't want to bother him further.

The doctor reaches for his script pad and begins to scribble.

"What are you writing? I thought you said referrals would be up front?" Mellissa asks.

He doesn't respond for a moment as he writes. "You asked me for Valium or was it Xanax? They're the same—like Coke and Pepsi. Anyway, I think you can use it because you also seem anxious. You just about tore out of your gown."

Who wouldn't be anxious sitting in a cold room butt-naked with a doctor trying to get out the door? And why exactly do I need to take my clothes off to have my heart listened to and eyes blinded? A simple, "Thank you," escapes her lips.

"If you want another opinion, you can find another doctor. And again, I will have the girls up front help set you up with a psychiatrist and fertility specialist. You can put your clothes back on now."

What the...? How many doctors does it take to screw in a light bulb or get me pregnant? Can they find out what is wrong with me? Do I have stress? Doesn't everyone have stress? She gets back into her running gear, fuming about the encounter.

Mellissa walks up to the front counter. Each stride feels slow and the squeak of her shoes on the clinic floor is aggravating her headache even more. Mellissa approaches the checkout counter.

"Mellissa, sweetie, are you OK? You look kind of pale. Did you have blood drawn?" asks Dawn, the receptionist.

"Damn it!" Her knees buckle and her muscles wobble like gelatin. She manages to reach a chair and sits down.

"Doctor! Doctor!" Dawn cries out.

"She's OK," says the doctor, materializing from the hallway. "She's a little anxious. Let's just make sure she didn't hit her head."

Heat creeps up her face and her heart races from embarrassment. "I am so sorry. I get this way when I miss a meal." The color floods back to Mellissa's face.

"You shouldn't skip meals," says her doctor, examining her head. "Anorexia is a very common sign of depression and it is also a common cause for anovulation. Here are the psychiatry and fertility referrals." He hands her the papers along with a handout labeled *Sleep Hygiene Instructions.*

"I was planning on going for a run through Centennial Park."

"But you didn't. Anhedonia. It's when you no longer enjoy the things you once did. So you avoid it. It's one of the top signs of depression. That and insomnia," he says. "Girls, get her one of the lollipops we give out to the kids after shots and bloodwork."

Mellissa wants to pull her hair and scream loudly. Just the thought of bloodwork makes her feel queasy again, but it isn't as intense as her anger.

"You have your color back," Dawn says as she hands her a red lollipop. "Oh, my! Now you're almost as red as the lollipop. Do you need help to the car?"

"No. I'll be fine. I just need some fresh air." Mellissa scurries out the door. As soon as she walks out, she leans against the door. *What just happened?*

She recaptures her breath and once the dizziness fades away, she starts walking to the car. She looks down at her Valium prescription and ponders whether or not to take it to the pharmacy. She decides to call Jez to discuss it.

"I need to rant today!" Jez says when she answers.

"Still no 'hello'?" Mellissa laughs, taking comfort in the fact she's not the only one having a bad day. "I thought you were looking forward to having a woman doctor? What happened?"

"I made an awful first impression." Jez grunts in response. Mellissa hears the exhaustion in her voice. "I couldn't sleep before the shift. Even after taking the Valium. I finally ended up passing out on the couch, but I had to take a second one. I felt groggy and just stumbled. She probably thinks I'm an airhead."

"I'm sorry. That actually sounds worse than my experience today at my yearly physical. I told him I had been having trouble sleeping and asked for Valium. He assumed I was depressed and didn't listen to anything I had to say."

"Hey, I remember you said you felt rushed last year. I thought you said you were going to find a new doctor?"

"I've thought about it. He always ran a little late, but you understood why because he took the time to answer any question you had. He even scribbled diagrams on the white exam table paper. He used to be more personable."

"When did things change?"

"I remember at first he talked about his fiancée, how he was looking forward to getting married. His eyes lit up when he talked about her. I remember this because he said the honeymoon was going to be in paradise. When I asked him where, he said, 'Paradise: The Island of Kauai.'"

"Ha!" Jez says. "You never told me that."

"His personality seems to have changed over the years. First, he stopped talking about his fiancée. Then the appointment waits got longer and the visits seem more rushed. As much as I love the girls who run the office, I think it's time to change."

"Why did you ask for a sleep aid? I thought it was just the stress of not knowing if you were going to get the promotion keeping you up?"

"Maybe it was just one bad night. I'll hold onto the script. Besides, I'm about to go out of town anyway."

Paradise Sleep Pearls: What makes us drowsy? Our brain utilizes glucose for energy. Similar to how a car uses gasoline. Glucose is the gasoline of our mind. When glucose is used for energy, adenosine is the exhaust left behind. All day the exhaust accumulates in our brain and makes us exhausted when up past a certain time. This is the body's process of making us tired at night, and it is called the homeostatic process.

During sleep, the adenosine clears, relieving the exhausted

feeling. Sleep deprivation results in left over adenosine and leaves you feeling exhausted.

Amlaner, CJ and Fuller, PM, Editors. Basics of Sleep Guide, Second Edition. Westchester, Illinois: Sleep Research Society, 2009

Airport Trance

Mellissa stands on her porch watching the morning sunrise over the Nashville skyline. She sees the color on the nicknamed "Batman Tower".

Once again, she sleeps through her morning run. She feels maybe this proves she has forgotten how to sleep. *It is no longer just work-related.*

The one solace this morning is she made last night's insomnia as productive as possible. Instead of flipping through TV channels or scrolling through her Facebook feed, she spent the night packing her bags and catching up on work emails. *Maybe I can turn my curse into a blessing.*

"Ready to go?" Mellissa jumps slightly at Rick's voice.

Mellissa smiles. "I didn't think I would see you today."

"You know I'm always your chauffer to Nashville International Airport." He grabs Mellissa's carry-on luggage as he eyes her. "That is a colorful outfit."

"The designer is from Spain. He originally made his way by coloring shirts by hand on the streets of Barcelona. He was so popular he ended up opening his own line. See, it says Barcelona on the shirt. You like it?"

"You look like a Zumba instructor."

"Ha! Let's go, funny man. The expressway is not so express at this time of day."

Mellissa doesn't mind the long drive—as long as she's the passenger. She enjoys sitting back and looking at Nashville's rolling hills. The small talk with her husband lets her mind wander during the pauses in their conversations. It's never awkward and always relaxing.

"When is the last time you talked with your mother?" he asks.

"It has been well over a month, actually. She has been in Central America."

"I know she's always wanted you to go with her. Why don't you do that sometime?"

"I didn't go this time because I was working so hard on the promotion. The timing just wasn't right."

Time passes on the highway without even one thought of the road. Mellissa daydreams about fond times she had growing up with her sister Dedee and her mother. Mellissa's trip down memory lane transitions into thoughts of the flight as she sees the signs for Nashville International Airport in front of them. They pull into the drop-off area and her husband parks the car.

"Listen; please get your snoring checked out while I'm gone."

"I told you, I don't snore."

Mellissa pulls out her phone and shows him a video of the snoring she made a few nights before. "Man Up! Get yourself taken care of." She knows nothing gets under a man's skin more than a girl telling them to "Man Up."

Rick looks up at her and smiles in affection. "OK. OK. I'll make an appointment with my doctor." He gives her an almost humorous look. "But you know I can't wear one of those masks. I don't even like scuba diving because of breathing through that stuff." Rick gets out of the car and helps Mellissa to the curb with her carry-on bag. "I remember when they used to let me walk you to the gate."

"Looks like you will have to get your goodbye kiss here."

Rick looks her in the eye. He smiles and bites his lip. He puts each hand on her waist as his thumbs move in a slow circular pattern around her panty line and says, "I love you." He pulls her in just a bit closer, pausing for just a moment as he continues to stare into her eyes.

It drives her crazy, in a good way. "Even after all these years, you've still never kiss me the same way twice."

"It's because I love you more every day." He takes his right hand and moves her hair behind an ear. The back of his curled fingertips brush her cheek just below the eye. They both tilt their heads and their lips meet.

A moment goes by and they pull back, looking at each other. Mellissa smiles. "I love you, too. I don't mean to be so moody, especially when I haven't slept well."

Her husband takes a step back. "It's OK. We'll work it out. Congrats again on your promotion, boss lady."

"Thanks," she says, smiling at him one last time before turning around and walking toward the sliding glass doors. She eyes his reflection in the glass until she walks through and passes it by.

Mellissa takes a straight shot through the airport. She is literally in a trance. The only thing on her mind is getting to the gate and sitting down so she can read her new romance novel.

She gets through security quickly and checks her phone. She finds a text from her husband: Already missing you Mel Honey.

Mellissa's trance ends when hearing the last call for flight 345 to Los Angeles.

Her seat on the plane is next to a dad and his three-year-old boy. Mellissa sits down and hopes the kid doesn't throw a tantrum. The boy looks at her as she gets her stuff together.

"So do you have any kids?" asks the father.

Not wanting to get into it, she looks down at her hands and says, "No."

The awkward silence is eventually broken when the father says to the boy, "Let me read you a story."

The father pulls out the emergency pamphlet from the seat pocket. "Once upon a time there were people on a plane..."

The boy interrupts his father, points to the flight attendant demonstrating placing a mask in event of a cabin pressure change and says, "He's putting on a CPAP, just like Grandpa!" Mellissa chuckles.

She tunes out the rest of the flight attendant presentation as she can recite it herself from the amount of times she has heard it and reaches for the airplane magazine. As she feels the rumble of the plane rising, she flips through ads for sleep pillows including a cumbersome wedge pillow that she has never seen anyone use on a plane. Her ears suddenly pop, signaling the plane is up. She continues to flip through the pages of the magazine. An advertisement for Paradise Sleep says: *Take a sleep vacation in the paradise of Southwest Florida and receive a professional sleep analysis by a Behavioral Sleep Medicine Specialist.* The ad goes on. *Medications are not first line therapy for insomnia! At Paradise Sleep, we offer Behavioral Sleep Medicine as non-medicinal approaches to a peaceful night's sleep.*

Guaranteed to help you sleep better with our five-session plan or your money back.

"Wow," she says, tearing out the ad.

She feels something warm on her left arm. Looking over, it's the little boy's head.

"I'm sorry," says the father.

"It's OK," Mellissa says. "Let him rest." Inside, she says, *Romance novel time!*

As soon as she gets into the book, she hears a ding, followed by the flight attendant saying, "Fasten your seatbelts and put up your trays in preparation for landing."

She opens her eyes and realizes she fell asleep. "Here already? I don't even remember closing my eyes."

"Yeah, you were out cold as soon as you started reading. You must not find the book interesting," the father says.

"No. I love the book. I guess I've been so stressed for so long that I crashed." Mellissa looks at the advertisement for Paradise Sleep, sitting in the open V of the book in her lap as a bookmark. She closes the book.

"I never understood why they're so strict about the trays coming up," he says. "It's almost as if the wheels of the plane are connected to the trays and the wheels won't come out unless they are all up."

Mellissa laughs, dropping the book in her purse. When she looks out the window, she sees the green land as the plane dips toward the airport. Mellissa takes her phone out once the plane lands. This time she has a text from her husband with an image attached. It's a picture of the pregnancy test. It is negative. Mellissa looks down and sighs as her shoulders drop.

Paradise Sleep Pearls: Our sleep wake cycle is also called our circadian rhythm. Indeed, it consists of a sleep phase, a wake phase and there is a transition between sleep and wake. The sleep phase occurs as a result of a combination of melatonin release at night in combination with the fatigue from the homeostatic process.

Although we live in a 24-hour society, in the absence of environmental time cues, the average free-running human circadian cycle is just over 24-hours. Phase shifting occurs when time changes occur (such as daylight savings) or during travel to different time zones.

Lee-Chiong, T. (2010, August) Circadian Rhythm Sleep Disorders. Sleep Medicine Board Review. Orlando, FL

Tennis Anyone?

Deciding to go out to dinner with Rick upon her return, Mellissa feels the strain of jet lag from being in different time zones and once again, fatigue creeps in.

They open the doors to the restaurant and hear the shriek, "You're pregnant!" The whole restaurant freezes and everyone looks in the direction of a couple sitting with what looks like two of their parents.

"Do you want to go somewhere else?" Rick asks as they walk up to the hostess.

The young hostess smiles at them. "Just the two of you? Any children?"

"Come on, Mel, let's go somewhere else instead." Rick tugs at Mellissa's crossed, stiff arms.

Mellissa's ears heat up as she musters a smile for the hostess. "Yes. Just the two of us tonight."

"Great! You must have a babysitter." The hostess takes two menus and heads toward the restaurant floor.

"No babysitter," Mellissa snaps.

"Oh, I'm sorry. I mean…I'm sorry you don't have kids. I mean…I'm sorry I misunderstood. I'm not sorry you don't have kids. I mean…," The hostess flounders. They reach their table and stand awkwardly around it.

"I apologize." Mellissa shakes her head as she waves her hand toward the hostess. "I didn't sleep at all last night. I get snippy…but we're celebrating tonight."

"Oh, wonderful! Is it your anniversary?" asks the hostess,

quickly regaining her perky natural demeanor and balance.

"Nope," Rick interjects with a beaming smile. "Job promotion. She's the boss lady now."

"Congratulations! I could see how that would keep you up at night. I have the opposite problem. I put my head down on a pillow and I am out. I can't even stay awake through a movie." The hostess laughs.

Mellissa gives the hostess a blank stare. Rick jumps in. "What was all the commotion about a minute ago?"

The hostess smiles. "It's graduation at the university today. A couple who just graduated found out the wife was pregnant two days ago."

The hostess walks away as the waiter comes by with water and to talk about the menu. Mellissa sees the waiter's mouth moving, but he sounds 100 feet away. The only thing Mellissa hears over the sound of plates, silverware and distant voices is the mother of the young husband on her phone calling one friend after another and yelling, "I'm going to be a grandmother!" and, "Yes, she's finally pregnant!"

Finally? Mellissa's mind drifts. *They just graduated. That seems odd…most people would be happy if their kids waited a few years after graduating to get married, let alone pregnant.* Mellissa feels the waiter tug at her menu. "Wait, we haven't heard the specials yet," she protests in confusion.

The waiter pauses with confusion on his face. He looks at Rick, who uses his hands gently to pry her fingers from the menu. "Mel Honey, I just ordered for you. He did tell us the specials and I ordered you the surf 'n' turf. I know you love Maine lobster."

Mellissa lets him take the menu from her. Embarrassed, she looks at the waiter.

"She didn't sleep at all last night," Rick tells the waiter, who nods and walks away. "Mellissa, honey, I know we talked about dinner and going down music row, but I think we should just have dinner and call it a night."

"I'm so sorry. I'm just exhausted. I get a little bitchy when I feel this way. My mind feels like it's filled with the dark exhaust from a construction truck."

"I thought it was the job promotion keeping you up at night. Is there anything else on your mind?" Rick asks.

"Nothing is clear to me right now. I do have the appointment with the fertility specialist tomorrow. Maybe we'll get some answers and that will clear some things up."

"One thing is clear to me." Rick releases her hand and reaches to his pocket, from which he pulls out a tiny turquoise box with a bow. "I'm in love with the boss lady."

Mellissa smiles and looks up from the box at him. "What is this?" Rick shrugs his shoulders, then points twice with his chin at the box in a "just open it" gesture. Mellissa's eyes sparkle as she opens the turquoise box. "You are so funny," she says, taking out a tennis bracelet. Her head tilts from side to side as she examines it.

"They still haven't invited you to play tennis, huh? Not even after the promotion?" Rick asks.

"They never do," she says wistfully. "They never will invite me into their boy's club."

Rick smiles. "I have to tell you, now that you've gotten the promotion—I was worried about your future with them, too. I know how much it bothered you when you gave a killer presentation and then Barry received a pat on the back and invited to play tennis or golf with the guys."

Mellissa laughs.

"Mel Honey, you have no idea how much I have felt your stress over the last year. You're not the only one who stayed awake worrying. I would actually long to hear the fire bell go off so I wouldn't have to think about it in the middle of the night."

"Not to change the subject, but now that I've gotten the promotion, why don't you stop working at the fire department and do your saltwater aquarium business full-time?"

"You know I can't do that."

"I know, I know, you will always be a fireman. I just worry about you, too."

Paradise Sleep Pearls: Jet lag occurs when one's internal circadian rhythm remains aligned to the home time zone and not synchronized to the new local time zone. Symptoms can be sleepiness in daytime and diminished alertness, as well as insomnia at night. Symptoms may be more pronounced with eastward travel that requires one to advance their sleep time. Generally, it takes approximately one day to adjust for every one-hour time zone changed.

It is important to note one does not necessarily need to "travel" to feel these effects of time zone change. When one has irregular sleep and wake times from week to weekend, essentially one changes time zones.

Lee-Chiong, T. (2010, August) Shift Work and Jet Lag. Sleep Medicine Board Review. Orlando, FL

Fertility Clinic

This time Mellissa has socks on so she is not cold in the paper gown. Mellissa sees a mirror on the wall to her right and looks into it. *Mirrors are really hard things to look away from*, she thinks. Her body looks skinny but doesn't feel like it as she puts her hand on her belly and pats it. She doesn't understand why she has a belly bump despite having thin arms. *Maybe I need to do more abs.* She lifts up her arms and looks at them. *I wish my arms were toned. That would make my little black dress look so hot.*

Mellissa flexes and says in a deep voice, "Strong is the new skinny." The doctor knocks at that moment and walks in while her arms are still flexed in the air.

"OK, Linda Hamilton, here comes the Terminator. Do you want me to come back later," he says in a relaxed tone. Then he adds in a poor Austrian accent, "I'll be back!"

"No, no. Sorry. I know you must be busy." Mellissa blushes.

"Busy?" The doctor pauses for a moment. "I am here. If my mind is elsewhere, thinking about what other things I have to do, then indeed we can call that busy." The doctor smiles back to Mellissa. "How can I help you? How long have you been trying to get pregnant?"

"We have been trying for about two years but stopped trying to prevent it about two years before that. I have tried everything I have read in *Cosmo* and on the internet, different positions and different boxers for my husband. I read about fertility drugs and hoped you could prescribe some. My doctor told me you could get me pregnant. As awkward those words were." *Although, with that bad accent, maybe he does father*

40

many children.

"I am not against medications. I frequently use different fertility medications. But let's just say I am more into looking into what we are actually treating. There are many different reasons for anovulation. Some may not be related to you, but may have to do with your husband. Before we start running a number of tests and conducting procedures, we need to get a sperm sample. But your husband's sperm is just one possibility for why you're not getting pregnant. There are many others. How is your sleep? Do you smoke? What's your calorie intake?"

"I think my calorie intake is fine. I eat three meals per day and snacks between meals. However, my sleep is awful. I never sleep. I just can't sleep at all. What does that have to do with getting pregnant, though?"

"Well, there are different hormonal releases that occur when you sleep. Chronic sleep deprivation or shifts in your sleep and wake cycle can cause anovulation. This was actually discovered in a large study done on nurses working the night shift. It found that night shift nurses were much less likely to get pregnant than day shift nurses. So I think this is where we should start, with better sleep."

"Well, my doctor gave me a script for Valium. I hadn't filled it yet, but I guess I will."

"Actually, you are going to have to do this without medication. If you are planning to get pregnant, we can't expose the baby to any medications. They may cause birth defects."

"I can't sleep without medication. I can't even sleep with the over-the-counter medications that I have taken in the past."

"Mellissa, I would advise that we find out why you are having difficulty sleeping. Before running fertility testing and considering treatment options, we should target your sleep problems first. Sleep difficulties are more common in women and there are treatments."

"I'm sorry, but I don't understand." Mellissa shifts uneasily; putting her palms up and further enquires. "You're recommending we treat my sleep first, but you said we can't treat it because of the risk of birth defects."

"Good question and actually rather common. Not all treatments involve medications."

"But I have already tried melatonin and natural options."

"There is a growing field of what is called Behavioral Sleep Medicine. When I was in medical school, our sleep lectures consisted of merely sleep medications. However, sleep science has evolved into its own field. Just like there can be many reasons why a person is having fertility issues, there are also many reasons why a person has difficulty sleeping. Maybe you would benefit from seeing a sleep psychologist."

Wow. Mellissa remembers the advertisement she saw for Paradise Sleep.

The doctor continues, "There are many excellent reading sources that are coming out on this. However, an experience that I have had is that there are many reasons for sleep problems. The cliché, one size fits all, is not always true."

"I understand now and actually I believe I know of place where I can find a behavioral sleep specialist. I'll look into it when I get home."

"Excellent! What about the other question. Do you smoke?"

"I rarely ever smoke."

"That means you do smoke." The doctor pauses for one moment and empathetically smiles. "Look, I'm not judging. People who smoke go through a lot of prejudices and we are all people with different habits. But if you smoke and take hormone treatments of any type, you are at increased risk for blood clots. Remember our goal is pregnancy. If you do get pregnant and have a baby, you risk a higher rate of SIDS."

Mellissa suddenly feels overwhelmed. Her expectations were one simple treatment for fertility. She was not expecting other issues needing to be addressed, especially ones she feels no control over.

"This is a lot to take in at one time. Can we work on the sleep first?"

"Absolutely." Her doctor smiles. "I am here for you. When you feel you want to proceed with evaluation just let us know. I will let you work on the sleep aspect first. And if you want to proceed with your husband's sample, we can do that as well."

Mellissa exhales. "I appreciate it. I feel more relaxed taking one step at a time."

"I understand. Do you have any other questions?"

"Not about fertility."

"What else can I help you with Mellissa? You seem to have a question on your mind."

"Is your office slow today? I mean, you've taken a lot of time with me. I appreciate your explanations. The last doctor I went to seemed rushed and commented on how there are not enough hours in the day."

Her doctor laughs. "Our schedule is full. I just believe that if we as doctors take the time to make sure the patient understands, there will be less questions in the future. And there will be less unnecessary testing. And as for having more hours in the day, I've always said to myself that if I had more hours in the day, I would still be right here, right now."

"I have no other questions. Thank you." Mellissa smiles. She decides to go straight home and talk with Rick about the appointment.

Paradise Sleep Pearls: There are complex effects of sleep and circadian rhythmicity on luteinizing hormone, follicle-stimulating hormone, and estradiol in women. Evidence suggests shift work is associated with menstrual irregularities, reproductive disturbances, risk of adverse pregnancy outcome and sleep disturbances in women. Sleep disturbances may lead to menstrual irregularities and changes in menstrual function.

1. Amlaner, CJ and Fuller, PM, Editors. Basics of Sleep Guide, Second Edition. Westchester, Illinois: Sleep Research Society, 2009
2. Labyak S, Lava S, Turek F, Zee P. Effects of shift work on sleep and menstrual function in nurses. Health Care Women Int. 2002 Sep-Nov; 23(6-7):703-14.

Say What?

"Say what! They want me to do what in a cup?" Rick grumbled.

"I told them you wouldn't be able to do that."

"No it's OK. I can do that for you. You do know I would only do it for you."

"Um, OK. Thanks?"

"No worries Mel Honey. I love you."

"Do you do that kind of stuff when I am not around?"

"I have no idea what you are talking about. Personally I think this is a waste of time because I'm not shooting blanks."

"So I'm the problem?"

"What? I didn't say that."

"You sure implied it!"

"Mel Honey, I'm sorry. Look, you were gone for a few days, now you're telling me to go rub one off in a cup. I'm just a little overwhelmed."

"I'm sorry. It's a lot for me to take in as well. If you don't want to go through with it, I completely understand."

"Will they have *Cosmo* there? Or do I have to bring one of your romance novels?"

Mellissa considers grabbing a *Cosmo* and smacking him with it. She pauses while she plays the scenario in her head, her hands twist as she envisions rolling up the magazine.

"Mel Honey, I'm just kidding."

"Ha!" Mellissa gets up and walks away with the first excuse

that comes to mind. "I need to make a phone call."

Mellissa wasn't aware nurses working night shifts and sleep-deprived had fertility problems. *Could that be my problem too*?

Mellissa looks for her novel in the bedroom. She wants to read and just get away. She finds her novel and lies in bed to read it. She finds the advertisement she was using as a bookmark, Paradise Sleep.

Initially feeling relaxed after walking out of the fertility clinic, she now has anxious thoughts again. *I have to quit smoking. I have to read a handout on sleep hygiene to be able to sleep. I have to sleep to get pregnant, but I can't use any meds because we are trying to get pregnant. I can't do this on my own. I need help.*

Mellissa considers searching for the script her doctor wrote, though she doesn't remember if it was for Xanax or Valium. *I guess it doesn't matter if it's Coke or Pepsi. Then again, if they are both the same and it doesn't matter, why do I even need medication for sleep?*

Feeling the need to blow off steam, she throws her running gear on and heads out of the bedroom to go for a run. On her way out, she takes every *Cosmo* from the house and puts them all in the recycling bin.

Paradise Sleep Pearls: Never go to bed angry.

Couples in heated discussions commonly fall into three categories regarding their communication– those who digress into threats, those who avoid the conversation resulting in silent fuming or sarcasm, and those who speak openly and respectfully. When emotions crank up, certain brain functions shut down preparing to fight or take flight. Taking time alone allows your body to calm, so you can then think clearly and compassionately. Coming to agreement to discuss topics later is not the same as avoidance.

Patterson, K. Grenny, J. McMillan, R. Switzler, A. Crucial Conversations, Tools for Talking When Stakes Are High. Second Edition. McGraw-Hill. New York 2012

Paradise Sleep

Mellissa again tries to take advantage of the time awake in bed by answering work emails. Caught up with work, she makes the ritual gravitation to the couch. Rick left early to work on some aquariums. He had put a pot of coffee on before he left and Mellissa detects the scent of morning coffee. *My elixir of life.* She drags herself to the kitchen.

Feeling fatigued, she pours a cup of coffee and sits at the breakfast table with the laptop. She decides to look up the Paradise Sleep website. Pictures pop out at her. Pictures of happy families, babies sleeping and kids sleeping in costumes. One really catches her eye. A maternity picture with the caption: Sleep and Pregnancy.

Great! I can't sleep now and if I ever do get pregnant, I'll sleep worse? She reflects on the problem her sister has. *And what about a baby crying? Dedee always complains she needs to wake up in the middle of the night to rock the baby back to sleep. She has to sing her a different song each time.*

Mellissa wonders how badly she really wants to get pregnant. *Maybe not everyone is fit to be a mother.* She continues to surf the Paradise Sleep website. Sleep Retreats.

Hmm. I've heard of yoga retreats. I've flown to a few cities to run half marathons. And there are couples' retreats, weight-loss retreats, even anti-aging conventions. I guess it's not that radical of an idea. And I always sleep best when I travel.

Mellissa dials the 1-800 number. She feels she has nothing to lose, yet worries she may lose her husband if she can't conceive due to a lack of sleep. No matter how often Rick says the idea is ridiculous, the fear is real to her.

"Thank you for calling Paradise Sleep. I'm Cindy. How can we help?" A female voice answers. Though the voice is perky, it doesn't sound like a young teenage voice.

"Hi," Mellissa replies and pauses for a moment. "I saw an advertisement about a sleep retreat."

"Yes. It's a five day retreat in Sanibel, Florida. We help people with insomnia learn how to sleep without the use of sleep medications."

"So how exactly do you guys treat insomnia without medications?"

"That is a great question and the root of the word question is quest. That is why it is a five day retreat."

"Fair enough." Mellissa shifts in her seat uncertain.

"If you pull up the website for the American Academy of Sleep Medicine, you can see the practice parameters for insomnia yourself."

Mellissa quickly types in the name and finds the site.

"It states that first-line treatment for insomnia is behavioral sleep medicine." Something else catches Mellissa's eye while Cindy goes over the information. "And if a sleep medication is started, it should be done along with behavioral sleep medicine interventions."

Mellissa is intrigued. "I've never even heard of behavioral sleep medicine."

"And if that hasn't captured your attention yet, I can show you multiple studies that sleep aids, regardless of the kind, work within the first two months but lose effectiveness at around two years. In fact, there are studies of people given a sleep aid or behavioral sleep medicine as therapy. It's been shown behavioral sleep medicine therapy was just as effective as medication in the short run. And at two years, the medications seemed to lose effect but the people who used the behavioral sleep medicine techniques had improved insomnia scores."

Mellissa smiles when Cindy refers to herself as the "day coach." All the information is overwhelming and heading to Sanibel Island to spend five days there gives Mellissa a lot to think about.

Cindy's warm voice continues, "Once a day you'll have a session with a sleep therapist in the afternoon and each morning there are physical fitness and beach activities."

"This sounds perfect since I'm also looking to tone up." Mellissa laughs.

"There is also ample leisure time as well. Most people use it as a vacation."

Mellissa figures she wouldn't have to take actual vacation time off because she mostly works from home.

"If your sleep has not improved in five to six weeks—then no payments. There are also no up-front payments. You just give a credit card number that gets billed if the sessions were helpful."

"Say what!" Mellissa shrieked. "If I sleep well, I keep my job and my marriage, for less than what a fertility evaluation costs? When can I start?"

"You can start tomorrow if you want. All our sessions are one-on-one. The summer is a flexible time around here. Fall and winter are busier with people in the north looking to get away from snow."

Without discussing it with her husband, Mellissa gives her credit card number to Cindy and agrees to the five-day escapade in paradise. After she gets off the phone, Mellissa receives an email survey from the clinic that she's supposed to fill out prior to arrival. She opens it up to find several forms, including a separate survey of what appears like endless questions, each with a: If yes, explain why.

Mellissa looks at question one. Does it bother you if you can't sleep?

What kind of a question is that? Of course, it bothers me. She checks yes.

Now for the "If yes, explain why" part. She types: If people couldn't stand the thought of not sleeping even when they're tired and know that it's going to make them a zombie the next day, then this sleep retreat wouldn't exist!

I'm not quite sure what I just signed up for. This survey should actually just be one question: Do you sleep, yes or no? Feeling desperate, she fills out the entire survey.

She then buys her plane ticket online and starts to pack her suitcase. She calls Rick to let him know she starts sleep therapy the next day.

Paradise Sleep Pearls: Caffeine counteracts adenosine. Remember that adenosine build-up in our brain causes fatigue and sleepiness. This is one way it makes you alert, but also a reason why if you drink caffeine late, one is not tired for sleep at night.

Amlaner, CJ and Fuller, PM, Editors. Basics of Sleep Guide, Second Edition. Westchester, Illinois: Sleep Research Society, 2009

Palms in Paradise

"I'm not in Nashville anymore," Mellissa says as she walks out of the plane upon arriving at Southwest Florida International Airport. Clean white shell tiles line the floors and walls. She hears the clank of her heels as she walks. There is a different feel to this airport. One of the first airport shops she sees sells bikinis, swimsuits and sunglasses. Another gift shop has Florida sweets, rum cake, coconut bars and orange cake. "The orange cake looks good," she says and keeps walking. Big glass windows allow the blue skies and Florida sunshine to pour through and light Mellissa's path to the car rental kiosk.

Mellissa exits the airport's main door and stands at the crosswalk waiting to cross. She catches a whiff of saltwater. She looks around but doesn't see a beach or a fountain, just tall royal palm trees all around. "Tropical doesn't describe this place," Mellissa says.

"Paradise does." Mellissa hears from her right. A tall, thin, old man with long white hair in a ponytail and a Santa Claus-like beard is standing beside her. He has a faded Tommy Bahama shirt and sandals on. He says, "Sorry to startle you. When you get to be my age, you lose your filter for interrupting conversations, especially when you see someone talking to themselves. Though that gets confusing nowadays, since people appear to be having conversations with the air, but it turns out they have a tooth gadget in their ear."

"Bluetooth," Mellissa replies.

"No, none of them are blue."

Mellissa smiles, wanting to correct him, but doesn't. She notices his tropical shirt must be one of his favorite shirts to keep wearing it after years of washing and drying. "I like your Hawaiian shirt. Have you ever been there before?" Mellissa asks.

"Someone special gave it to me years back," he says with a smile. "Funny how everyone calls it a Hawaiian shirt. I always viewed them as Florida shirts. This is how people dress here. Even the fanciest restaurant here, where proper dress is required, Florida shirts qualify as proper dress code."

Mellissa laughs. "Well, I like your dress code and it sounds like you know your way around the restaurants here. Is there a place that makes regional deserts?"

"Oh goodness, yes! The diabetic industry should have their headquarters here with all the old people and sweets," the old guy replies. "My name is Sam and it's not every day that I run into a young pretty girl. Actually, it's more like every other day."

Mellissa laughs again. "Hi Sam, I'm Mellissa."

"Calamondin Cafe. I actually heard you say that the orange cake looked good as we were walking past the gift shop. Best orange cake you can imagine. Calamondin Cafe."

"Cala what?"

"It's a type of orange; small and more tart and citrusy than bigger oranges. If you can't pronounce it, just call it an orange. So what are you doing here? I take it you're not visiting family since you're going to the rental car and asking about local places. I make good observations, don't I? Do you need help with your bags?"

"I'm on some kind of sleep retreat. Have you heard anything about those?"

The old man starts to laugh. "Lawrence. He knows his sleep. You'll be fine."

Mellissa isn't sure why he is laughing and doesn't like to be laughed at. However, the laugh seems reassuring–if that even exists. "Lawrence?"

"Yeah, he's a crazy son of a bitch." Sam laughs.

Mellissa gulps. "Great…" She shakes her head.

"Good crazy, though. Don't get me wrong. He gives community talks all the time around here. You will be fine. Just don't ask him about his dog. That is the one thing he rambles on about," says Sam.

"Appreciate the tips." Mellissa nods her head in a goodbye gesture as she looks toward the car rental place.

"No worries, sweetie. Have fun and sleep well in paradise."

Paradise Sleep Pearls: Most age-related sleep changes occur in early and mid-years of the human life span. Sleep efficiency decreases as aging continues. Consequences of disturbed sleep may include attention problems, slow response time, memory and performance problems, all of which may be misinterpreted as dementia. There is an increased risk of falls in elderly sleeping less than 7 hours per night and increased risk of mortality in elderly sleeping less than 5 hours per night.

Gooneratne, N. Sleep Disorders in the Elderly. Board Review for The Sleep Specialist Course. 2009. American Academy of Sleep Medicine.

Sleep Retreat Session #1:
I'm Not Psycho

Mellissa walks into Paradise Sleep. There is a small waiting room, no receptionist and a few scattered magazines.

Mellissa looks around the room. In one way, she expects to see diplomas everywhere. Instead, she sees pictures of children. The children are awake, sleeping, dressed liked fruit and sleeping in odd places, like musical instruments and airplanes. The photos are beautiful and unique.

"Like the décor?" comes a voice behind her. Startled, she looks back. A tall man with a runner's slender build and a light dusting of salt in his hair is standing there. He is wearing a tropical shirt with palm trees. Something is on his nose, right on the point, but she can't make out what it is.

"Sorry," Mellissa says, blushing.

"For what?"

"Oh, I was just looking at your portraits. They're so beautiful. You must be the sleep therapist?"

"Were you expecting someone different?"

A simple yes or no would have been fine. She keeps trying to make direct eye contact, but her eyes keep drifting back to his nose. She feels like the guys with elevator eyes when she wears her bikini at a pool.

"I find the ones of the kids sleeping, relaxing just as I find the ones of the kids awake and playing to be invigorating. Do you have any kids?"

That question again. She swallows trying to get the lump out of her throat.

"My name is Lawrence. I assume you are Mellissa?"

"Yes, I'm Mellissa. Nice to meet you, Lawrence." Mellissa feels relief not having to answer the question, but embarrassed to be so transparent.

"No need to be embarrassed about anything. We'll work through anything we can during these next five days."

That was weird. I guess I must wear my emotions on my sleeve.

"Let's get started. Come into my office." He leads her through the door and down the hall to a large, modestly lighted room. There is a desk and large leather chair with a tall back, but there are also several other chairs and what appears to be an antique couch like the stereotype of what one sees in a psychiatry office.

"Is that an old psychiatry couch?" Mellissa continues to try to make eye contact, but his nose is between his eyes. Instead, she decides to look at his right eye only.

"I'm not exactly sure what a psychiatrist chair is, but I am not a psychiatrist. Sometimes people need to put their feet up, they usually do it when they are not as guarded."

Mellissa chooses not to sit on the couch, but rather a cushioned chair next to it. "Um, OK, what exactly are you? My doctor gave me a referral to go to a psychiatrist."

"Why?" Lawrence passes his desk and sits in a chair across from Mellissa.

"Well, I told him I couldn't sleep so he told me I was depressed." Mellissa looks at the floor.

"Did he ask you if you felt depressed?"

"No, he just assumed that is why I couldn't sleep. And I tried to tell him that I'm not depressed."

"Hmm. Typical. So tell me, what are the things that are bothering you?"

"I can't sleep. I have tried everything. Well, not everything. My doctor gave me a script for Valium, but I never filled it because..." A feeling of failure overcomes her. *I can't bring up trying to get pregnant.* She continues, "Because I saw your ad in a magazine on a plane about Paradise Sleep and thought I would give it a try."

"Plane magazines are entertaining. I have yet to see a dweeb sleeping in that clunky giant inflatable plastic pillow. I swear, if I ever see a person using one, I will take a picture of it and post it on Facebook."

Mellissa laughs. "I had the exact same thought the other day!"

"So you told me why you are here, but you didn't answer my question. What are the things bothering you?"

"Excuse me?" Mellissa is baffled by the question. *Why else would I be here?* "It bothers me that I can't sleep. Why do you ask that? Do you see other disorders besides sleep?"

"Who knows?" says the therapist. He pauses for one moment then repeats himself but more slowly. "Who knnnooowwwsss?"

Busted! I must be staring at his nose. She feels the heat of embarrassed again. The urge suddenly to get up overcomes her. The heat on her face must be turning it red by now and her body tightens.

"Mellissa, I have gone through your questionnaire and it seems like you have a certain level of psychophysiological insomnia."

"I'm not psycho!" A defensive tone echoes in her voice.

"Good, because I am not a psychiatrist. I think we established that. I am a behavioral sleep medicine psychologist and I see a lot of this."

Mellissa's muscles relax. The notion her disorder has a name and Lawrence has seen a lot of it gives her hope.

Lawrence smiles and Mellissa feels he knows he has her attention. "You see, commonly people can't sleep because something is on the mind. However, what is on the mind is that the individual can't sleep. Have you ever seen a dog chase its tail?"

"Well, yeah. Don't all dogs chase their tails?"

"Not Pembroke Welsh corgis. They don't have tails. I once had one. Everyone kept asking me if I cut my dog's tail. I replied, 'why on earth would I cut my dog's tail?'"

"Excuse me, but can we talk about your dog later?"

"I used to have a dog, but I don't have one anymore."

"What happened to it?"

"I thought you didn't want to talk about my dog? It is frequently on my mind but let's move on. Yes, you have seen a dog chase its tail, but you have never seen a dog actually catch its tail, right?"

Not sure if she should be confused or happy he knows exactly what is going on with her, Mellissa raises her eyebrow and frowns.

"Again, and hear me out, you have difficulty sleeping because something is on your mind. What is on your mind is that you have difficulty sleeping. You try so hard to sleep that you think about it. However, the more you think about it, the more it keeps you awake. We call this psychophysiological insomnia."

Lawrence reaches to his nose and peels off what appears to be a piece of masking tape with red marker on it. Mellissa can see that underneath the tape his nose is fine. *Why would he go through such a charade?*

"You saw something was on my nose. You kept looking at it. The harder you tried not to look at it, the more your eyes kept coming back to it. Almost like when you're in high school and you have a crush on a guy—the more you think about him the harder you try not to look at him, but you always seem to get caught glancing at him. And heaven forbid you have a pimple in high school. Everyone tries to look away, but it always seems like they keep staring at it. Just like when I get lettuce in my teeth..."

"OK. I get your point."

"Great! Is anything else bothering you?"

"I told you that I can't sleep."

"OK. Then we are done for today." He gets up and brushes away the folds from his khakis.

"What? That's it? What happened to the five days of sessions? Over just like that? I booked a room here, you know."

"The five days are still on. It's just that we are done for today. This first session is used to find out about things that are bothering you."

This bothers me! Mellissa shakes her head and sighs.

Lawrence smiles and sits back down. "You see Mellissa, insomnia is a symptom. People can't sleep for a reason. Sometimes they have anxiety, sometimes they may have a medical disorder, such as restless legs syndrome or sleep apnea. Or there could be physical pain keeping you up. Frankly, the psychophysiological insomnia part of your sleep troubles is just the tip of the iceberg."

"That makes sense." She never really thought about "what" was keeping her up. "I assumed it was simply I was incapable of sleeping." *Or my husband's snoring.*

"I approach insomnia as one should approach weight management. Lifestyle and habit changes are stronger than the power of a pill."

How does lifestyle influence sleep? Mellissa feels the expression of a deer in head lights creep upon her face.

"And then, Mellissa, we frequently develop life-threatening events that keep us up at night. Life-threatening doesn't mean you will get eaten by a lion."

"How dramatic." Mellissa laughs at the notion.

"The stress of your job, getting fired, getting married and worries about infidelity all threaten the way our life is as we know it to some degree. Not having children..."

"I really don't want to talk about that. I am here to get help with sleep."

"Mellissa, I don't view insomnia as an isolated night disorder. There are things happening all daylong that contribute to your problems with sleeping at night and if you don't sleep, well you feel the effects the next day. Insomnia is a 24-hour disorder."

Mellissa's eyebrow rises and the frown returns.

"Mellissa, what would you like to talk about?"

"Well, I was referred to a psychiatrist to find out what was wrong with me." Lawrence raises his finger and goes to speak, but Mellissa quickly says, "I know, I know, you are not a psychiatrist! My doctor gave me a printout for sleep hygiene. How come you didn't list that in your advertisement?"

"Because sleep hygiene is crap."

"What?"

"Mellissa, have you even looked at the paper? I mean you haven't asked me specific questions about any of its content. You just say that you got handed a paper."

"I saw there were ten topics."

"Ah, yes! The proverbial ten commandants of sleep. Handing someone a list of instructions for sleep doesn't work. Let me give you a different example. Let's discuss weight management again."

"I'm confused. I'm here to talk about sleep, not weight management."

"Correct. What I am trying to do is give a different example of instructions versus explanations. For example, it's not helpful to give someone a list of instructions for losing weight. If you tell them, don't drink soda, they go home and drink juice instead. It needs to be explained that the sugar content in a soda is equal to that of juice. The sugar content of juice may be equivalent to four to five whole pieces of fruit when it takes only one apple or orange to satisfy you."

"Then what does work?"

"Understanding the basics of what occurs when you are awake and asleep is actually one of the most powerful things that will help you sleep. Again, insomnia is a 24-hour disorder."

"Curious." Mellissa shifts in her seat.

"I am curious, too, Mellissa. I am not trying not to bounce around. But I am curious as to what things are bothering you. During the day, at night—within your entire day. I understand it may be difficult to talk about. We will go at your pace." Lawrence reaches for an iPad on a nearby table, makes a note and places it back.

Mellissa has many ideas in her mind about the things that bother her. She wasn't expecting to discuss any of them on this trip. Her expectations were more along the lines of lists of do's and don'ts about sleep. If she knew she was going to end up thinking more about her infertility, smoking and pressures from her husband and their family then she would not have signed up for the sleep retreat.

Mellissa takes a deep breath, holds it in for two seconds and exhales slowly. This always seems to relax her and help her to move forward before talking about difficult topics.

"Well, like you noticed by my pause earlier, we don't have any kids. We've actually been trying to get pregnant. My younger sister has two children. My husband wants children."

"But do you?"

"What?" Mellissa hadn't really thought about it. "I mean, I like our time alone. I like our travels to Paris and wine country. When I look around here, the beaches are so beautiful, but they are so loud with kids. And I really don't like minivans."

"What else is bothering you?"

"My husband wants me to quit smoking."

"But do you?"

"Not really. I don't have a problem with it. I only smoke one cigarette a day and I run almost every day. But when my husband looks at me, it's as if I'm just a pair ovaries. I can see in his eyes that he's picturing my uterus shriveling and coughing from the smoke. I don't need to see him frown and shake his head at me."

"So, Mellissa, here is a different question. You say you don't want to quit. But do you feel you could quit?"

"Oh, definitely. It's not crack. I could quit cold turkey if I wanted to."

"If you wanted to?" Lawrence says.

"Which I don't."

"When did you start smoking?"

"In college. I went backpacking through Europe with my friend Jez. We flew in through Paris first. It was just common to smoke there. It's not unusual to sit at an outdoor café and see your waiter in the street with his back turned as if he suddenly can't hear, smoking a cigarette. We had a lot of down time, you know, waiting for our waiter…so I gave it a try and I liked it. After that summer, when we returned home, I would hang out with my friends. We would smoke. It was something to do. I like how it feels. Everyone else was smoking with a couple of drinks."

"So in college you started smoking daily?"

"No, not daily. Just when I had a few drinks with friends."

"When did you stop limiting it to only with drinks?"

"Well, in grad school, I had an intern position. Oh my goodness! I don't want to talk about that. Do I have to?"

"No. You don't." After a moment of silence, Lawrence says, "I'm just trying to figure out what truly bothers you as opposed to what is bothering others. Just wanted to know how things developed."

"Well, during my internship I had a romance with a guy that I worked with. That was his name actually, Guy. He was smart. We got along and worked well together. He told me he was divorced and had what looked like a fresh tan line around where his wedding ring was. We would take extended lunch breaks and go back to my place. We would have great sex. Then we would have a cigarette before we would part ways so we could arrive back at work separately. It was fun while it lasted, but it just didn't work out between us."

"He probably would have ended the romance early if you didn't smoke, just as you would have lost your college friends if you decided to quit. And you probably would have never enjoyed Paris if you didn't take that first smoke."

"What? That's ridiculous."

"Maybe." Lawrence crosses his legs and makes another note on his iPad. "So, at first you just tried it, later it was something to do with drinks and then something after sex. By the way, the affairs in the daytime, was the sex in bed?"

"What kind of question is that? Yes. Of course." Mellissa doesn't want to go into the different places they had sex in.

"My apologies, but you'll have to trust me when I say you will understand my question in the future, just not today. So when did you start smoking casually?"

"When I couldn't sleep."

"Something to do?"

"Yes. Not sleeping when you want to sleep is boring. The thought of being in bed awake irks me."

"Psychophysiological insomnia. We will work on that later. Do you still smoke after sex? I mean I am assuming you still have sex, otherwise that would be why..."

"OK. That's enough." Mellissa adjusts her position in her seat and crosses her legs.

"Let's digress from sex. You say your husband doesn't like it when you smoke. So you must smoke in front of him."

"No. I wait 'till he is asleep. If I can't sleep when he's asleep, I go out on the porch to smoke." Mellissa pauses.

"Tell me how that goes," Lawrence prompts her.

"Well, I put on clothes; then I go onto the porch. I smoke one cigarette furtively. I put it out with the dew on the porch. But if it's not dewy, I put it on the sidewalk, go inside and get some water so I can pour it on the butt to make sure it is out. I don't like to flick the butts on the ground where he will see them the next day. Then I bring it to the bathroom and flush it down the toilet so he won't see it. I then wash my face and hands. Sometimes I take a shower if I feel like I still smell. Other times I'm exhausted and just light a scented candle."

"Exhausted? How long does it take to smoke the cigarette?"

"Less than a minute. I rush through it and don't even usually finish the whole thing."

"How long does it take to put on clothes and then clean up?"

"I don't know? Two, three minutes? Five maybe? I haven't timed it."

"Wow! That seems like it's a lot of work to continue doing something you said you could quit cold turkey. Do you feel as if you are addicted? Have you ever had to use a nicotine patch or chewing gum?"

"No."

"Makes sense. Some people call nicotine use a pseudo-dependence or a soft addiction. If you were able to sleep through the night, you would go anywhere from seven to nine hours without it. People don't just wake up and light a cigarette in bed either. They usually get up and make their coffee first. Now you say you have traveled to Paris, that's commonly an overnight flight without nicotine. You're right; it's not crack. Your words."

"Let me guess, you are telling me to quit too. Just use my will power? Don't expose my baby to it, if that ever happens."

"Why would I ask you to quit? I asked what is bothering you and you didn't say smoking is bothering you. Actually, you said it was bothering you that your husband wanted you to quit. And you didn't say that not getting pregnant was bothering you. What I heard was that other people are bothering you about these things. I don't mean to put words in your mouth, but that's what I heard."

"What does any of this have to do with sleep?"

"Remember, we're looking at your 24-hour process, Mellissa." Lawrence pauses and picks up his iPad and pushes his finger on the screen.

"What are you doing?"

"I apologize, Mellissa. I need to take notes from time to time. I also want to take a moment to set, not so much a goal, but rather a vision. Give me a vision statement about your sleep."

I don't even know what that is, I'm no Mensa. Mellissa feels the conversation is jumping around. Now also confused about what bothers her as opposed to what bothers others. She takes another deep breath, holds it in for two seconds and speaks her mind. "My goal is to sleep."

"I know what your goal is. But so far, what I have heard is, 'I cannot sleep.' Let me give you a parallel example. If you give a kid of cup of milk and say, 'don't spill it', they will literally visualize themselves spilling it and they get nervous. However, if you give a kid a cup of milk and tell them how proud you are they are holding it carefully with two hands, they don't visualize a problem and they enjoy the milk more."

Mellissa laughs. She sees a picture in her mind of her nieces and nephews squirming in their chairs at dinnertime and their father saying, "Don't fall and crack your head!"

"A vision statement is the first step in restructuring your beliefs about sleep. It is actually not unique to sleep but as you stated, that is why you are here. I want to take a moment now to set a vision statement."

"OK. I am going to be able to sleep someday. I can't do it now but that is why I'm here."

"Not so fast. The word 'going' is a process not a vision. You currently visualize yourself as unable to sleep and you believe you have no control of it. Don't spill the milk. We are in the process today and through the rest of this week of teaching you how to hold the cup of milk gently. To sleep well, you need to visualize yourself as able to sleep well. It starts with a vision statement. Here are my rules. One, your vision statement needs to be in the present tense. Two, focus on what you want, not the process of what you want to move away from. Three, no negatives."

"OK. I will..."

Lawrence quickly interjects, "'I will' is in the future, but your vision statement needs to be in the present."

Mellissa can't see herself sleeping. She sees herself tossing and turning. She thinks, *don't spill the milk. What does milk have to do with sleep?* Unsure if there is anything to the whole warm-milk-and-sleep thing, Mellissa remembers as a child she often went to bed at different times, sometimes on her own and sometimes not until her mother came home. On those occasions, her mother would give her that warm cup of milk. It seemed to help her rest. *And that was the last time I actually rested peacefully.* She returns to the present, where she's supposed to give a vision statement. "I have restful and peaceful sleep every night."

"Good statement." Lawrence smiles.

"That's it? I just had to make a statement and I'm now cured of my insomnia? You could just put *that* on your website."

"It's a process, Mellissa. During this five day retreat, you are going to learn a sleep diet—that just means lifestyle changes for better sleep. You're going to meet with me in the afternoons and with Cindy in the mornings. If you are nice to her, she'll also take you shopping."

"Shopping? What does that have to do with sleep?"

"A lot actually, I assure you shopping will help you sleep."

"I'm game."

"For today, what can I possibly tell you that is going to make you sleep? Nothing. In fact, I have learned more I say in one session than less is learned because you are fatigued and sleepy from your insomnia. Insomnia is a bitch—I get it. I once struggled through it. Most of us do. Even before our 24-hour global society made these problems worse, insomnia was present. Before Ben Franklin ever flew his kite to discover electricity, the Scottish had a term called 'agrypnia' that meant insomnia. I kind of like the term agrypnia better actually." He then repeats it a couple of times, as if experimentally, in a bad Scottish accent. "*Agrypnia!* I can't sleep because of *Agrypnia!*"

Mellissa laughs. "So you don't have a magic bullet?" Trying to bring him back to the topic at hand.

"What I have is an axe. And with it we will chip away at the contributing factors to your insomnia over time."

"An axe? Nice male metaphor Paul Bunyan."

Lawrence gets up once again and brushes off the wrinkles in his pants as he did earlier. "We are going to call it a day for now. You are learning well, but it is time for you to meet up with Cindy so you can plan out the day activities."

Mellissa is surprised and relieved. She wants to go on and learn more, but is at a point where her attention is fading. She gets up, grabs her strappy handbag and starts to head toward the door she came in from.

"Hold on Mellissa, come out this way instead. I like to respect people's privacy so I have a different exit."

Lawrence walks Mellissa through a different door that enters into a hallway with a different exit. As they pass through the hallway, Mellissa sees another room with the door half cracked. The room is dark, but just as it is dark, it is equally vibrant in colors. Mellissa peeks her head in and sees two large saltwater marine aquariums. Brain coral, sea anemones and a medley of drifting fishes with every color in combination that one can find in a crayon box.

"My husband Rick loves saltwater aquariums."

"That is my meditation room. It is my place of mindfulness." Lawrence opens the door at the end of the hallway for Mellissa's exit.

Mellissa raises one eyebrow higher than the other as the crease between her eyebrows wrinkle. "So if you can't sleep, you get up and go back to work to relax?"

With a warm grin, Lawrence replies, "Actually, relaxation takes practice. This is where I practice. And when it takes me a while to sleep, rather than coming here, I envision myself here. I envision the tranquility of the collage of colors, buoyancy of the ocean water, surrounded by the warmth of darkness. It allows me to drift into a peaceful nights rest."

Mellissa nods as she heads out the door. "Thank you."

"I will tell Cindy you are on your way."

Paradise Sleep Pearls: Agrypnia was originally described as a vigil before certain feasts, the rite of staying awake for devotional purposes.

In The Study of Medicine in 1822, Agrypnia Excitata is described as irritative wakefulness, sleep retarded by mental excitement. It also stated, "The cure of this species of sleeplessness is to be accomplished by allaying the mental excitement by which it is produced."

Agrypnia pertesa was described as chronic wakefulness, sleep retarded by bodily disquiet. Examples provided of such bodily disquiet included aching coldness, uneasy stomach, hunger and "if those who are accustomed to wine at night take tea instead they cannot sleep." Once again, "The cure of this disease demands on particular attention to its cause."

Good, JM. The Study of Medicine. Baldwin, Cradock, and Joy. London. 1822

Tiki Bar

Mellissa walks up to the Harborside Resort, which has an old Key West style exterior with local tropical flora. *I'm in Florida.* Mellissa walks in. The sliding doors open and a whoosh of air-conditioning makes her shiver for a brief second, but it feels good compared to the humid day. She passes the dark coconut palm wood furniture and the poolside captures her eye. She walks through the lobby and feels the air circulating from the large Tahitian like fan blades on the ceiling. Entering the poolside, Mellissa feels the humidity again and detects the scent of a well-kept clear pool. The scent is aromatically mixed with a blend of coconut from suntan lotion as well as the fruitiness from the banana daiquiris being mixed at the bar.

Mellissa walks up to the dry palm tiki bar and approaches the bartender mixing drinks. A mid-sized man, lean with his hair straight back, however, naturally flowy. A thick Italian accent takes Mellissa by surprise. "Signora, what can I get for you?"

"You're not from around here are you?" Mellissa smirks.

"I am from Naples."

"Hmm. Naples is less than an hour away. I wouldn't have guessed you had an Italian accent." Mellissa sits at the bar.

"Naples, Italy. My name is Palo." He removes a yellow hibiscus flower in a miniature vase from in front of her and places a cocktail napkin. "You are already a flower. The bar can only hold so many beautiful flowers at one time."

Mellissa wants to laugh because his response seems so stereotypical, however instead she blushes as he expressed it so genuine. "Did you say your name is Paolo?"

"No, it's Palo." He then spells his name, "P-A-L-O. What can I make for you?"

"A Florida drink. Surprise me."

"Sí, signora." Palo turns and grabs a long clear glass. He squeezes lime juice into it, puts a dash of sugar and then places fresh mint leaves in the glass. He uses the back of a spoon to crush the mint leaves. Then he adds sparkling water. Bubbles fizz on the mint leaves as he gives them a second grind. He adds white rum from the bottle, just eyes it. Then he counts as he adds ice cubes. "One, two, three, four, five and six. Just like Hemingway would have daily."

"Excuse me? Are you Mellissa?" Mellissa turns to the woman's voice just beside her.

"Yes. Are you Cindy?"

"Yes, I am. Welcome to Southwest Florida. Nice to meet someone else from Nashville."

"Buonasera Cindy." Palo pops the cork of a wine bottle and pours Cindy a glass of red wine.

"Buonasera Palo." Cindy takes the glass of wine and Palo walks to the other side of the bar to a group of laughing girls just arriving.

Mellissa hadn't known what to expect. She is surprised to learn Cindy is from Nashville. Her mental image was of a girl with a lisp like Cindy from the *Brady Bunch*. Cindy instead was of medium height, with a friendly smile and a physique like the one Mellissa wants. Her blonde hair fit nicely with her slight tan. Cindy's fashion style was trendy and complimented her physique by showing the definition in her shoulders.

"Did Lawrence do the knows/nose thing?" Cindy smiles and takes a sip of her wine.

"Ugh! Yes. You mean to tell me he does that all the time?" Mellissa did an eye roll.

"Some of his psychology colleagues have said it's unprofessional. He says that it's unorthodox but nothing else seems to make a lasting impression for him to make his point about how psychophysiological insomnia can build over time. He says that before he started using his knows/nose technique; patients would just keep saying over and over again that they weren't psycho. Besides, all those forms you filled out before you got here help make sure that your sleep is not affected by a different mood or medical disorder."

"So tell me, Cindy, what is your part in this deal? Other than Lawrence telling me I need to be nice to you so we could go shopping."

"Shopping is therapeutic and there's a whole lot of shopping around here so you can have as much therapy as you want."

Both ladies laugh.

"My role is to exhaust you daily so you sleep well at night."

Mellissa didn't know if she actually liked the sound of that. The thought of massages and occasional running on the beach sounded more appealing.

"I have degrees in psychology and counseling. But I'm also a certified personal trainer and I own my own CrossFit gym. So Lawrence and I are kind of like yin and yang."

Not exactly sure what she signed up for, Mellissa ponders having arms like Jillian Michaels and getting sleep all in one. But a "Day Coach" going full Jillian on her wasn't part of the plan. "I don't know if you need to exhaust me. I actually sleep well when I am traveling. Especially when I can hear the ocean hitting the beach. It's at home where I cannot sleep."

"And as long as you believe that, you won't."

Mellissa's eyes open-wide. "Excuse me?"

"Lawrence does the knows/nose thing with everyone. He also doesn't let people leave the first session without coming up with a vision statement. What is your vision statement?"

"I have restful and peaceful sleep every night. That is my vision statement."

"Nice. Now what do you currently say to yourself at night when you don't allow yourself to sleep?"

That's an odd way to put it. When I don't "allow" myself to sleep? She must have no idea what it is like to have every racing thought of the day spin through her head while feeling pure exhaustion. I'm a victim to insomnia, not its cause! Mellissa frowns, crosses her arms and says, "Insomnia is a bitch!"

"That's a new one. Can I tweak that just a touch?"

"Go ahead, Coach."

"Insomnia is a beach." Cindy pauses and smiles for a moment. It's not a smug smile but rather the same type of nurturing smile Mellissa's mother would have on her face when she gave Mellissa a glass of milk as a kid. "Go along with what we say. There will be activities. There will be sessions. There will be times that you are tired, times that you have energy you never thought you had. There will even be some experiments. And when the time is right...there will be shopping."

A certain level of trust flows through Mellissa in response. *Seems like they know what they're doing. If their plan is so good, why would there be an experiment?*

"To quote Picasso, *'Everything you can imagine is real.'* And you will learn to imagine yourself sleeping well and it will become reality."

"But tonight, we have our cocktails. Cheers." Mellissa raises her glass and then takes a long sip.

Paradise Sleep Pearls: People who exercise frequently report better sleep then those who don't, even when both groups get the same amount of sleep. Regular exercise may reduce anxiety more effectively than many antianxiety medications. Exercise also improves sleep because the physical stress on the body causes the brain to compensate by increasing its deep sleep.

1. National Sleep Foundation Poll Finds Exercise Key to Good Sleep. Sleepfoundation.org
2. Jacobs GD. Say Good Night to Insomnia, The Six-Week, Drug-Free Program Developed At Harvard Medical School. Henry Holt and Co. Holt Paperbacks September 2009

Sunrise High

Mellissa loves to look out the balcony of a hotel room with a sunrise beach view while she holds her cup of morning coffee, but not today. Instead, at 5 am she had the choice of CrossFit or a sunrise jog on the beach. She chose the jog, not realizing it meant getting up early to drive to Bowman's Beach on Sanibel.

Mellissa hears a knock. Followed by Cindy's muffled voice chiming, "Knock, knock!"

Just one would have been fine. Mellissa opens the door and immediately notices Cindy wearing the newest Lululemon. "I love Lululemon!"

"Me, too. We get the newest stuff here because we have a Lululemon store at the Waterside Shops in Naples. Don't worry. It's on our agenda."

They get into Cindy's car and head over the Sanibel Causeway. Daylight begins to break and just enough light outlines the structures on the island ahead. As they drive onto the island, Mellissa notices an old rustic lighthouse on the left. To the right there are million-dollar homes. "That is a lot of house to clean."

Cindy chuckles. "And you know you can't afford it if the thought of an expensive electricity bill is the first thing that comes through your mind."

"Coconut trees and hammocks in the front yard. Amazing that people actually live here," Mellissa says. Wonderment glues her eyes to the old style Florida homes with plantation shutters, dogwalks and warp around balconies. Soon the scene is replaced by Periwinkle Place shops, a set of boutiques and art galleries. "Chico's!"

"Yup. That is actually the original store. I'll tell you what; we can hit those on the way back. After we cool down and have breakfast at the Blue Giraffe, that is. They have this panwich that is so good—its two fresh eggs with ham sandwiched between two pancakes. Yummy!"

"I'm game. No arm twisting." Mellissa's stomach rumbles at the thought.

"Are you a talker? Some people when they jog, all they do is listen to their iPod. Others like to talk. I can do either. Lawrence is an iPod person. He always complains about how he needs new music 'cause he is tired of the same songs, but he doesn't like to listen to any modern music. I flipped through his iPod once and he had the 'Humpty Dance' on there."

Mellissa laughs. "I'm a talker. I can run on my own with an iPod but when I run with someone, I like to run 'with' them. I like the interaction."

They arrive at Bowman Beach. Dawn is starting to break, but they have flashlights with them as they walk towards the beach. They cross over a short bridge that carries them over a saltwater marsh before reaching to the beach. It's not long enough to loosen up the joints, but it is long enough for Mellissa to relax into the tranquility, the mangroves and the many different kinds of birds.

Cindy sets down a cooler with sports drinks, bottled waters and bananas. They do their stretches and start out with a light jog.

"I noticed your attention goes to the birds. Sanibel has one of the highest varieties of species of wading birds: herons, ibis, osprey, anhinga, cormorants, pelicans and so many more."

"I find it peaceful," Mellissa says. "I can't wait 'till the sun is fully out so we can watch them soar through the sky. How can you tell them all apart when they are so far in the air?"

Cindy nods her head. "Good question. You can't always see their feathers, beaks or talons from afar. Much of bird identification is based on impression: the way they glide, how they beat their wings and at the way they look from different angles.

These all form patterns. We all form patterns, actually—you may recognize someone you know without seeing their face because you notice sequences of different struts and mannerisms that are unique to them. It's the same with birds. They each have unique bird movements that combine to create what cannot be described in words."

They continue to run as the sun gradually rises. Mellissa sees the color of the shells on the beach rather than just feel a slight crunch as they step on them. Mellissa feels each step on the beach takes a little more work and requires slightly different muscles than the hills of Nashville. At least she doesn't feel the jarring on her knees and hips like she does when she runs on the sidewalk around her neighborhood. "Running on sand is different. Where I live there are hills. Going uphill I generally have short steps and my head is up looking at the crest of the hill as I try to keep my posture."

Cindy smiles. "It *is* different. It's a more intense workout on different muscles. Beach running at first can feel like you have weights on your ankles."

"I notice it is harder to plant my feet and equally a little harder to get each foot off the sand as well," Mellissa pants.

"This is real soft sand," Cindy replies with a bounce and a smile. To Mellissa it appears Cindy is accustomed to beach running. "In this sand your heel strike doesn't come down and hit a firm surface. Instead, your body adjusts by relying on the muscles around your ankle to keep the foot steady. And because the surface is not flat, your foot can't go flat either. Your calf muscles help work to normalize the motions. We will have to stretch those well at the end with a foam roller."

Mellissa intended to talk with Cindy on this run, but feels winded. The feeling of her heart pumping while seeing the colors of a sunrise is majestic. Mellissa takes a deep breath of the ocean air. She feels great. "Normally when I run, I look at the hill crest or a light post, or count the number of houses. But out here, I see the ocean to one side, palm trees and sea grapes on the other. I keep seeing this paradise unchanged."

Cindy smiles. "It is as if time passes without any evidence that time has passed. That's why I wear a watch."

Eventually it is time to turn around. Mellissa has no idea how long the run back will be since she doesn't know how long they have been running. The sound of the ocean is in tune with the feeling of her blood flowing. With every few beats of her heart, she becomes aware of her endorphins. Her mind feels connected to her body and she feels the soft tingle of pins and needles around her back, shoulders and even her cheeks as they brush with the salty wind. As her body experiences the rush, her mind becomes more alert and sharp.

"Impressive! I like it!" Mellissa says on her runner's high.

"Some people have extreme experiences with beach running. My mind is always more clear during a beach run and more relaxed after. The feeling is indescribable to words. I once had to write a paragraph about what a cantaloupe taste like. No words did it justice. My friend Rena came closest. She described it as an orangey, peach colored, sweet, slippery, juicy flesh that melts in your mouth, ripe with a dampened sweetness."

Mellissa's mouth waters. Cindy's analogy had nothing to do with running, but she understands that some things are better experienced then explained.

"By the way, we are done with the run."

Mellissa stops dead and puts her hands to her knees, panting. Her muscles become idle but her heart continues thumping her chest wall.

"We have to keep moving, though, you don't want to cramp up. Your body got a great workout, now we need to let our heart recover and balance our minds as well." Cindy turns around and walks backwards looking at Mellissa as she continues.

"Our minds?" Mellissa stands upright and takes steps towards Cindy with curiosity.

"Walk backwards with me."

Mellissa catches up to Cindy and starts walking backwards.

Cindy puts her arms out with her palms to the sky and looks up. She takes a deep inhalation through her nose and smiles.

"Aren't you afraid you are going to walk into something?" Mellissa asks.

"You mean like a giant squid? How many things did you dodge or duck under on this run?" Cindy still looks up at the sky.

Mellissa quickly realizes there's nothing but beach in her world at this moment so she mirrors Cindy's posture and looks at the sky as well, walking backwards.

"That's right." Cindy smiles. "I like to look up at the sky as the sun begins to rise. It is a great way to start your day, mindful with your environment. Our environment can influence our body through our nervous system. This is such a serene environment, it can influence your body and mind to a calmness."

Mellissa's mind clears. "I like what I am feeling but don't know what I am doing."

"Walking backwards uses muscles in the back part of your body. It balances your body. But equally it balances your mind." Cindy continues to walk, but instead of looking at the sky, she gazes straight at the beach and the shoreline. "Stepping back takes a conscious effort while you walk. Metaphorically, you look at where you have come from rather than being so focused on where you are going. I always do my best thinking when walking backwards."

Mellissa goes with it.

"There is so much stress in our society. Simple measures to balance our mind and body are often ignored. People talk about stopping and smelling the roses, but when you emphasize the stop, you re-emphasize that you have to go, go and go again. You can keep moving towards where you want to go in life but to take a simple moment to reflect on where you come from helps you to see exactly how far you have come. Otherwise, you will always be bogged with the stress of how far you still have to go."

Mellissa gives the understanding smile Cindy has been giving her. "Like now. I'm walking backwards, still moving towards our destination of our towels and water, but looking at this stretch of shore allows me to appreciate how great this run was."

Cindy reciprocates the smile.

Mellissa's mind tries to clarify where Cindy is coming from. Still unclear as to what exactly Cindy's role is. "Cindy, tell me your story. Personal trainer, sleep educator, day coach…I still don't understand."

"That is a long story." Cindy chuckles.

"This is a long shoreline and timeless too."

"Believe it or not I originally wanted to go into medicine. I was pre-med in college and I started dating a guy in medical school. We lived in Texas at the time. Financial ends were not meeting. My boyfriend helped get me a job as a pharmaceutical sales rep. Pharmaceutical companies know how to recruit girls that have enough intelligence to go to medical school, but also have family obligations that make them seek work. That is actually when I first was introduced to sleep. I worked for a drug company that made insomnia medications. You believe in what you do, believe in your product and believe that you are helping people. One day I went to call on a pain specialist and he suggested that I talk to a sleep doctor in town. Apparently, they were friends. I thought the sleep doctor was new, but the pain doctor told me that the sleep doctor had actually been in the area for five years. My first thought was wow, how could our company have missed that? I went back to my manager and looked into it, and there was no record of him ever prescribing any of the sleep medications. So I took it upon myself to call on the sleep doctor. I talked to him about my drug and gave him the data and the clinical studies that proved it was effective. He was very nice, but his response caught me off guard. He said, 'It might have a role in his practice.' *Might?* I really believed in what I did. I couldn't sell a product I didn't believe in. I pushed the envelope a little more and asked him, 'What do you mean by *might* and how come you haven't shown up on any of our company data if you have been here for five years?'"

Mellissa catches her ponytail swaying, only slower now they are walking. Her attention quickly shifts back to the story.

"The sleep doctor told me that he rarely starts people on sleep aids. I found that odd because he was a sleep doctor, what else would he do? He challenged me, asking if I really wanted to know. Of course! He bet me a million dollars—actually a lottery ticket—that my company has never shared with me the information that he was about to give me."

Mellissa raised an eyebrow.

"He went over the practice parameters for insomnia. Medication was not the first thing that was mentioned, but rather the behavioral treatments."

"That is the information you went over with me on the phone when I first called. I was amazed."

"I went home. I wasn't in tears, but felt emotionally zapped. I told my fiancé what I had learned. He told me he had never heard such things in his med school or residency training. He said that they had one lecture about sleep medicine, but it was about overweight men snoring because they had sleep apnea and need CPAP. He also said that in his psychiatry class they talked about sleep medication, but never really discussed what normal sleep was.

"Almost immediately, he was resistant to it. He said he didn't have the time to fish for sleep complaints in a fifteen-minute appointment. His last words on the conversation stung. I will never forget them. He said, 'Patients show up late, they show up early, they show up on time and they all show up at the same time and expect to be seen right away. There are not enough hours in the day.'"

Mellissa stops. "Those were the same exact words my doctor had said!" *It has to be the same person. What are the chances?*

Cindy stops and turns to Mellissa. "You OK?"

Mellissa keeps walking. "I loved the beach running. I'm just not used to it. I'll be fine. I think I just need to stretch my calves like you said."

"Let's go by the boardwalk and stretch there," Cindy says.

"I see your passion for sleep now."

"Yeah, I don't want to say that's what broke up our relationship. I ended up changing my major to psychology so I could be a counselor. We later moved to Nashville together. He got a good job offer coming out of residency. Then he started coming home later and later. It wasn't fun to be in a new place alone, without family. That's when I got into exercise and fitness. It was interesting as I continued my studies in psychology. It seemed to help me learn how to motivate others. It was a natural gravitation for me to become a personal trainer."

"That makes sense," Mellissa replied.

"Nashville is beautiful, but my dream was to live in a tropical paradise. I wanted to support him and I tried to put his needs over mine, but there came a time that we both realized we were trying to accomplish different things. Not to mention he wanted children, but I just didn't feel I needed that to make me complete. Our careers were growing, but our lives were drifting apart."

"Sorry to hear that." Mellissa tries to change the subject. "But you live in paradise now. I mean look around. People travel from all over to come to Sanibel."

Cindy's eyes start to water. "He always told me he would take me to paradise. We had purchased tickets to Hawaii. We were going to go to Kauai until I called off our wedding."

Mellissa feels several emotions at once. She turns to comfort Cindy.

"It's OK, Mellissa. I rebounded quickly. I actually met my husband shortly after that and we married later that same year. We moved into that relationship so fast that we had some struggles, but nothing that a true love couldn't overcome. Funny, though—I've never viewed it as a rebound, but really feel that I connected with my soul mate. Anyhow, it's in the past and it's part of what made me who I am today. I'm sure he has moved forward and is a better doctor today than I remember."

Mellissa opens and then closes her mouth. *Cindy still has a warm vision of who this guy is.*

"We had a great run, now let me show you some new stretches with this foam roller. Then we'll refuel at the Blue Giraffe."

Mellissa tries to say OK, but feels like her voice paralyzed within her throat.

Paradise Sleep Pearls: In a hallmark study by Morin and colleagues, the efficacy of sleep medications and behavioral interventions for insomnia were evaluated. Groups given an FDA approved medication and no behavioral treatment had short-term benefits, but relatively no long-term benefit. A group given FDA approved medication and behavioral treatment had better short and long-term benefits. Another group was given no medications, behavior treatment only. The study demonstrated the group given behavioral interventions with no sleep medications had better sleep two years after the termination of treatment.

Morin CM, Colecchi C, Stone J, Sood R, Brink D. Behavioral and pharmacological therapies for late-life insomnia: a randomized controlled trial. JAMA. 1999; 281(11):991-99.

Wall Nuts

The run went longer than either she or Cindy had expected. Though they opted not to go shopping at Periwinkle Place, they still stopped at She Sells Sea Shells since there are no shells in Nashville.

What am I doing here? Mellissa prides herself on her honesty. She knows Cindy's ex is now her ex-doctor. Mellissa obsesses about telling Cindy she knows her ex-fiancé. After all, people are linked in so many ways. How is this any different than looking at a person on Facebook who she doesn't know who shares 10 mutual friends with her? On the other hand, it would be insignificant if she decided not to say anything. Mellissa thinks about what Lawrence said.

"Psychophysiological insomnia: the more you think about something the more it becomes the source of the problem. Insomnia is a 24-hour disorder." Mellissa realizes obsessing over Cindy's ex-fiancé is no different than her own thoughts that won't let her sleep. Mellissa decides to take a leap of faith. She will learn how to do that over the next few sessions at the sleep retreat. *I'm not lying if I don't say anything about it. I mean, we know the same man but it's not like we both slept with him. And what is it with the sex questions Lawrence asked when we met? What does that have to do with anything? Sex in bed or sex on the wall, who cares?*

Mellissa didn't want to discuss details with Lawrence. The sex was indeed in bed when they started going to Mellissa's house during lunch, but then they would fall asleep and couldn't get back to work. Eventually they made it over to his house from time to time. There they never even made it to the bed.

Guy would rip her clothes off but in a way that never popped a button off her blouse. He pinned her up against the wall. He had an amazing way of kissing her neck as her silkiest underwear, worn for this purpose, came off. The feeling was beyond hormonal—it was an endorphin high.

Yes, now that she thinks about it, they always had sex against the wall at his place. In fact, Mellissa will never forget the first time they were making love against the wall. Right before she had an orgasm, he stated, "I love our wall nuts?" Mellissa immediately lost her focus as she about burst into laughter. At that very moment, he sent her into an orgasm like no other. *Damn it.* What do you do when your toes begin to curl—how do you keep from falling? She was saved as Guy grabbed each of her cheeks and supported her up against the wall.

It was more than the most exciting sex she ever had—it was the *best*.

What is the point of thinking about all this? Mellissa refocuses and feels confident in the Paradise Sleep regimen. *I need to focus on that.*

Paradise Sleep Pearls: Both men and women may feel sleepy after sex, though this is more pronounced in men. The act frequently takes place at night, in a bed and can be physically exhausting. Hormones have an initial influence on receptivity and later on sleep as well.

DHEA has an influence on readiness for sex and may give a natural amphetamine like high. In women, estrogen also influences receptivity as well as provides a softness. In men, testosterone peaks to sexual desire, lust. These hormones influence the initiation of the mating.

Oxytocin has been called the hormone of love at first site. There is a release of oxytocin with the touch of the skin. It gives a sense that your mate feels "just right". Oxytocin has been associated with bonding and equally has shown to reduce fear and good judgment. There is further a release in orgasm, which is believed to help reduce stress levels.

Orgasm also causes release of prolactin, which is linked to the feeling of sexual satisfaction. There is a link between prolactin and sleep.

For a person to reach orgasm a requirement is to lose fear and anxiety. This can be relaxing. Try it sometime. You may like it!

1. Gottman, J. Building Trust, Love and Loyalty in Relationships. CMI Education 2012
2. Kruger, D and Hughes, S. Tendencies to Fall Asleep after Sex are Associated with Greater Partner Desires for Bonding and Affection. Journal of Social, Evolutionary, and Cultural Psychology 2011, 5(4), 239-247.

Sleep Retreat Session #2: Sleep Restriction

"Are you crazy?" Mellissa asks Lawrence. "I am telling you I cannot sleep after midnight and you are telling me not to go to bed before midnight?" Mellissa grabs her purse as if she were about to leave. "There is no way I will be able to stay up that late!"

"You won't be able to stay awake? Then your insomnia is cured," Lawrence replies with his hands out and shoulders raised.

Mellissa feels her shoulders fall and drops her purse resignedly. *Lawrence has a point.*

"Look," Lawrence says. "You have had insomnia for over 10 years. I am asking you to continue having it for less than 10 weeks. And then it may be gone after that."

"You're saying sleeping less is going to cure me of my insomnia. You have to be kidding me. Are you sure this is going to work?"

"I am not psychic. In the phonebook, psychologist is listed just under psychic, but indeed, they are listed separately. I don't know when you are going to allow yourself to experience a peaceful night sleep. However, you are here. That tells me you're motivated. Well I'm motivated to help you! With both of us working together towards a common goal, I would say the chances are pretty good, huh? What do you think?"

"What do I think?" Mellissa mutters. She honestly thinks it has been two days now and this guy has still not yet answered a question directly. "Can you please say 'yes' or 'no' every now and then?"

"Maybe," Lawrence replies. "Remember, our sleep diet involves lifestyle changes."

"That makes no sense." Mellissa's ears feel hot to the rhythm of her pulse with his maybe response. "If I'm trying to lose weight, I need to eat less. My husband is trying to bulk up so he eats more. I can't sleep, which is why I have been spending more time in bed."

"And exactly how has that been working for you over the last 10 years?"

She breaks off eye contact and stares at her feet, focusing on the toe cleavage her marble red high heels provided.

"That's a cool bee tattoo on your foot," Lawrence says.

"It's a honey bee," Mellissa says finally, looking back up at him.

"A honey bee? All tattoos have an inspiration. Except for the ones that were alcohol-influenced and those are normally not placed in a visible area."

Mellissa blushes and looks down again.

"I asked you two questions," Lawrence says. "I thought I lost you for a moment, but now you have my curiosity with the honey bee tattoo."

"It's my name, Mellissa. My mother tells me that the moment I was born my father laughed and cried at the same time. She says the second he held me; he called me his sweet little honeybee. My mother had been reading on names and their meanings, and when she heard him say that, immediately, she named me Mellissa." Tears form at the rim of Mellissa's eyes.

"What does the tattoo mean to you?"

"I didn't grow up around him. He passed away when I was young. My younger sister actually doesn't remember him at all. What I remember is that he worked a lot. Both of my parents did actually. I tried so hard to wait up for him at night and mostly that was late because my parents ran a restaurant. I waited for him to tuck me in and he always said, 'Good night, my sweet little honey bee.'" Mascara ran off her face and smudged on her thumb as she wipes the tears away.

Lawrence hands her a box of tissues. "Are you sure your insomnia doesn't go back to childhood?"

Mellissa thinks back to her childhood. "I thought I slept fine. I was up late nightly but on weekends and during school breaks, I would catch up on missed sleep."

Lawrence starts to nod. "Hmm," he says, sitting up straight.

Mellissa's shoulders feel heavy as she exhales. "Look, I don't want to talk about my childhood to anyone. I am here because I can't sleep. I can't change things that happened to me in the past. I just want to know what to do so I can sleep well from here forward. I'm two days into this and don't see how getting less sleep is going to help me with getting to sleep at home."

"The best I can do is to find out how past events have shaped your current sleep habits. Understanding this will allow us to modify your habits and help you attain your vision statement of peaceful, restful sleep every night. After all, the best way to predict the future is to know your history."

Mellissa cracks up, tears stopping as she looks at Lawrence.

"I digress," Lawrence remarks. "Sleep diet. Let's use weight management as an analogy. There is no magic number of calories that a person needs to have. It all depends on the person and their goals. Let's say you want to lose weight and your boyfriend wants to gain weight. I wouldn't view it as you just eating less and him eating more. Rather, it is the content of the calories that needs to shift. In weight loss, one would reduce the fat in the diet, whereas in muscle building one increases the protein. Regardless, both people would avoid excess empty calories from carbs. You are not binge dieting, but rather changing your lifestyle. You engage in fat-burning cardio, while he engages in muscle-building power lifting. And by the way, the energy you expend during the day also leads to your night sleep drive."

"You lost me. Are you telling me to sleep more or to sleep less?"

"Well, look at it this way. You don't feel you sleep well now so if I told you to just sleep more that wouldn't be very helpful, would it? It's like when my son asks, 'Where is mom?' and I tell him to go ask his mother. It's just not very helpful."

Mellissa exhales with a quiet laugh.

"What I am talking about is time in bed, most specifically time in bed that we are not asleep. The more time you spend in bed when you are awake, the more it contributes to your problem of getting to sleep. The more you lie in your bed awake, the more you think about insomnia. The more you think about your insomnia, the more frustrated you will get about not sleeping—and in turn, that keeps you awake. Excess time in bed when you are awake is like the empty calories of sleep. Too many carbs will not help with weight loss and will actually contribute to unwanted weight gain. Spending excessive time in bed awake contributes to insomnia."

Mellissa nods her head.

"I didn't make this up. It has a name. It's called sleep restriction. It means that you restrict your time in bed to sleep time only. If you can't sleep, you need to get out of your bed and go somewhere else. And, regardless of what time you go to sleep, you'll have a strict wake-up time every day."

"OK," Mellissa agrees.

"There is no magic pill for weight loss. You can't sustain a healthy lifestyle with laxatives and binge diets. That is only going to lead into a cycle of weight gain after every period of weight loss. And then one day you'll stop trying because it always leads to weight gain anyway. Disparity sets in and people believe that they can't lose weight. Likewise, there is no magic pill for sleep either. Binge sleeping is going to allow you to get a regular sleep pattern. Lifestyle changes need to occur as well." Lawrence makes a quick note on his iPad. "Now, Mellissa, you revealed that as a child you would go to sleep late during the week and catch up on sleep over the weekend. How is that different than now? You don't sleep well at home, but you sleep great when you travel and your job requires lots of travel."

Mellissa nods.

"I'm more concerned about how you are going to sleep regularly ten weeks from now than tonight or ten hours or days from now."

Mellissa's tilts her head and squints, a perplexed expression on her face.

"So again, think of spending extra time in bed awake as being like empty carbs—they are both counterproductive. Our goal is for your sleep to be more efficient. And it is a myth that people need to sleep extra to catch up when they haven't slept well. When we are tired and fatigued from a night of poor sleep our brain and body rebound with more slow-wave sleep, our deep sleep and it occurs within the first four hours of sleeping. Our brain detects the fatigue, gets into a deep sleep quicker and is actually able to extend that deep sleep longer. So when we don't binge sleep, the depth and quality of our deep sleep are improved. That deep sleep is like the protein we need to build healthy muscle mass; weight management parallel again. Reduce empty carbs and eat moderate protein. In sleep we cut down on time awake in bed, cut down on excessive sleeping in and we allow our body to get into deeper more refreshing sleep."

"So by following your sleep diet, I will get more deep sleep—more REM sleep?"

"No, Mellissa. REM sleep is not your deep sleep. In REM, you dream, but that is a very active brain process and is not your deep sleep. We still have a lot to learn," he responds. "And no napping. Think of those as junk food for now. If you eat a candy bar before dinner, you aren't going to be hungry for dinner. Likewise, late naps or long naps, especially if they last more than two hours, interfere with getting to sleep at the time you desire. They interfere with your hunger for sleep, you sleep drive."

"That is the first time I have ever heard you say 'no,'" Mellissa remarks. "But everyone can have an occasional treat, right?"

"Yes…but if you are trying to lose weight, you want to establish your metabolism and lifestyle first. Then later, once your goals are met, you can introduce treats in moderation. And likewise with naps. No napping until we get you sleeping well regularly. After that if you want to nap on a hammock on the beach or on a rainy Saturday that is fine."

Mellissa is relieved she will be able to nap in the future. She enjoys a glass of red wine while watching the November rains from her window in Nashville. It usually leads to a nap with the soothing rumble of the thunder.

"And the most important thing is to follow a strict waking time. No sleeping in on the weekends. Think of sleeping in as the gristle on a steak or a buffalo chicken wing. Fat has nine calories per gram. It tastes good when I eat wings once a year, fried, then battered in hot wing sauce that contains butter and accompanied with a cold beer. But the next day, I feel so sluggish. Excess weekend sleep does the same. Sleeping in late, not getting your morning sunlight—these things can put you in a mental fog during the daytime and make it difficult to get back to sleep at your desired bed time."

"But if I don't sleep in, I'll be tired over the weekend," Mellissa argues.

"Are you suggesting that you should continue to sleep in on weekends, then not sleep well on Sunday night and be fatigued Monday morning at work instead?"

"Why can't you just give me a straight up set of instructions?" Mellissa pleads.

Lawrence laughs. "Like the sleep hygiene instructions that were given? I have come to learn that people with insomnia are tired and I am not being funny. People with insomnia are tired and no matter how interested they are in what I have to say, talking at you and not with you will eventually lead to drowsiness. Having you think through the problems will keep you mentally engaged."

"OK. So you didn't say you want me to be tired at night. You want me to use that fatigue to be able to get to sleep earlier the next day," Mellissa says.

"Yes!" Lawrence shows a proud grin on his face. "Now Mellissa, how do you feel? Do you feel more tired than you normally do at this time?"

"Actually I do, but it is because I woke up so early this morning for that sunrise jog with Cindy." Something occurs to her. "Did you plan that on purpose? Exercise first thing in the morning to make me tired?" Mellissa thinks about Cindy and how it was Cindy's job to exhaust her.

"It's unorthodox, but we have a plan. Tonight you will feel your sleep drive more than you normally do. It will help you get into a deeper sleep tonight. You'll see."

"I suppose if you had let me sleep in today, then I wouldn't be tired tonight and may even had some insomnia on my sleep retreat."

Lawrence leans forward and smiles. "You're making great progress. Let's call it a day."

They both get up. Mellissa leans to pick up her tissues. Lawrence beats her to it and grabs them.

"Oh! Don't touch those! They're covered in my mascara and tears and..."

"And your snot. It's OK. I have kids."

Mellissa laughs. She feels relaxed. He walks her to the door. As he shuts the door, he gives her a little nod to signal goodbye. Oddly, it doesn't feel abrupt.

Mellissa thinks Lawrence's approach is rather unusual, but she feels he is genuine. Lawrence is guiding, not tugging with her. She almost feels like they are walking down a path together and he is a step ahead of her trying to eliminate her down a particular side of the fork in the road. Mellissa feels empowered to make her own choices.

Mellissa begins to think about how to respond to Cindy's day lessons. She takes out her phone to call Jez in search of advice on how to talk to Cindy; however, it goes straight to voicemail, which states the mailbox is full. Mellissa shakes her head as she hangs up and sighs.

I need to tell her that I know her ex-fiancé. I'm not going to be able to focus on what she is teaching me if I keep trying to block out these thoughts. How am I going to learn to overcome my psychophysiological insomnia if I have psychophysiological in-learnia? Mellissa knows that isn't a real word, but it makes her smile inwardly.

Paradise Sleep Pearls: Sleep restriction is designed to consolidate sleep. The feature of this intervention is to reduce sleep extension.

A common misconception is to fall asleep earlier, one needs to get to bed earlier, sometimes several hours earlier then they plan to actually fall asleep. The process of being in bed awake while one waits to fall asleep is called sleep extension. Sleep restriction is an intervention to reduce sleep extension.

Perlis, M. Cognitive Behavioral Therapy for Insomnia. 2012, October. Bethesda, MD

REM is Not Deep?

Mellissa walks through the hotel and sees Palo at the tiki bar. Palo smiles and says, "Hello ladies."

Mellissa looks around but only sees herself. "It's only me, Palo?"

"I know, but you are twice the lady," he says with his Italian accent and smile.

Mellissa laughs. "How exactly does someone from Naples, Italy end up in Florida?"

Palo gives a half face smile. "Hmm. You would not believe it."

"Why wouldn't I believe you? Try me."

"What brings you here to the Paradise part of Florida?"

Mellissa didn't feel like declaring herself an insomniac. However, if random *Old Man Sam* knew about the sleep retreat then maybe it was more common than she had anticipated. "I'm here on a sleep retreat. Have you heard of it?"

"Of course!" Palo inflects in such a positive manner that it gives Mellissa hope. "Five day retreat, where you will learn how to allow yourself to sleep. You will walk out with visions of palm trees and ocean sounds as you lay your head to sleep once you leave."

Mellissa didn't know what to think, however, she feels reassured her problem is more common than she had imagined.

Palo replaces the cocktail napkin gathering beads of condensation from the humidity. "I tell you what; maybe I will tell you my story on day six."

Mellissa eyes Palo and gives him back the same half smile, knowing there is no day six of the five night retreat. She walks back to the lobby. She takes one last look behind her shoulder. Palo makes eye contact, gives her a quick wink, then turns back to his side to hand wash the cocktail blender.

Mellissa decides to call Rick before heading to her room. The phone rings a couple of times and right as Mellissa decides to hang up she hears, "How is my beautiful wife?"

She immediately exhales her worries. "I'm fine. I miss you."

"Wow! I don't hear that too often. What are they doing to you there?"

The Bluetooth she uses to make phone calls allows Mellissa to put both hands to her face, fingertips on her forehead and palms on her cheeks, she inhales and opens her eyes at the same time she says, "Oh, nothing."

"Nothing? You sound like a teenager, like my brother's step-daughter Samantha."

Mellissa's wishes she could sleep like Samantha. It has been the family joke to take pictures of her sleeping at family events. Mellissa views Samantha's life as peaceful and restful, except for the constant struggle with her biological father, who always calls her lazy for sleeping as much as she does. Rick's brother continues to insist there is a physical cause for her sleepiness.

"How is Samantha?" Mellissa enquires.

"Not good, actually, they are taking her to a psychiatrist because she started having hallucinations and passing out."

"Oh my! I hope she is OK. How have you've been? How is the CPAP?"

"Not good. I either wake up in the morning and the snorkeling equipment is on the floor or air starts to leak out of my mask and it dry tickles my eyes, waking me up." Rick quickly changes the subject. "Are you the only person there at the sleep retreat?"

"Yes, I'm the only one here. However, many people are familiar with it. What I have found surprising is there's a lot of talking about day activity and when to stay awake. I thought it was all going to be about how to sleep at night."

"You're at a sleep retreat and talk about being awake? Good thing they offer your money back. What exactly have you guys been talking about? And don't say nothing."

"I don't know."

"You really do sound like a teenager. How can you tell me it's a lot of talking, but then not know anything else? Come on Mel Honey, what is eating at you?"

Mellissa's mind swirls as she thinks of something legitimate to say. "Did you know that REM sleep is not your deep sleep?"

"Say what? Don't you dream in REM? How is that not deep?"

Mellissa never got an answer to that one. She needs to change the subject with something that will grab his attention like when her female friends start talking about a sale at Home Depot to their husbands. "Lawrence has this meditation room with these huge, beautiful, saltwater aquariums with all these colorful fish. He has clown fish, too."

"Aww! Were there any kids there looking for Nemo?"

"I so wish you were here right now." She looks away from the mirror and back down at her phone, which has his photo on the screen.

"Hmm." Rick's voice deepens and softens at the same time. "What would you do?"

Mellissa purrs, "I would…"

Just then, a loud siren goes off on his end.

This is why she hates to call him during his shift. She doesn't know if it is a house fire, arson or an apartment complex with a child trapped inside—who her husband wouldn't think twice about trying to save.

"Don't worry, Mel Honey. It's…probably another false alarm, probably the same kid pulling the fire alarm at the doctor's office. Happens all the time."

Mellissa looks outside and sees darkness. No doctor's office is open at this time. "Don't worry, huh? Don't spill the milk, either."

"What are you talking about, Mel? Look, I have to go. I'm sorry."

After they hang up, Mellissa takes her Bluetooth off and walks to her room. Even under the best of circumstances, in the finest, most relaxing hotel, she is going to worry about him and it is going to take some time to unwind.

Paradise Sleep Pearls: REM cycles

REM sleep is indeed our dream sleep. We normally don't get into our first REM period until about 90 minutes into sleep. And about every 90 minutes, we have another REM period. Each time the REM period becomes a little denser. The densest REM period is actually later in sleep, in the early morning. This explains why many times we remember a dream as our alarm clock goes off.

Our sleep cycles through the night between Non-REM and REM sleep. This explains why we may have more than one dream through the night.

REM is a very active brain period. During REM, we are consolidating memories into long-term memories. That is why you may have a dream of someone you haven't seen since childhood, but equally why you may have a dream of an event that just occurred the other day.

In REM sleep, our muscle tone is lower, almost like a paralysis. This protects us from acting out our dreams.

Amlaner, CJ and Fuller, PM, Editors. Basics of Sleep Guide, Second Edition. Westchester, Illinois: Sleep Research Society, 2009

Namaste on Captiva

Mellissa and Cindy head to Captiva Island for a yoga session on the beach. Mellissa spent the morning in the resort business area catching up with work emails. She is thankful it's midday when they start driving. The Florida sun is out in full force. This time around, in the light of day, Mellissa can actually enjoy the scenery as they enter the island.

They approach the Sanibel Causeway, where the Gulf of Mexico meets the Caloosahatchee River. Even though it's bright and sunny, there is a nice breeze guiding windsurfers as they rip through the water at fast speeds and glide through the air in a series of jumps.

"Check out that sign!" Cindy points to a wooden board with the outline of an alligator, with writing next to it.

"Don't feed the alligators. Oh, my!" Mellissa says.

"There's a large sidewalk through the island. It's big enough for a small car but made for bikers and golf carts."

Mellissa looks at the sidewalk, filled with people on bikes and foot. She looks around and sees something dark and suspicious, "Is that an alligator?" Mellissa anxiously grabs her pounding chest and her eyes open wide with a sense of alertness. "Sorry, it's just a log." She exhales slowly as her heart relieves and her mind relaxes.

Cindy laughs. "You should have seen it before Hurricane Charlie in 2004, around the time my husband and I moved here. There were these large banyan and mahogany trees that shaded the roads and sidewalks. People would sit out in their Adirondack chairs but now they need to look for a place under a tree in their yard rather than just anywhere."

Mellissa doesn't say much. If she asks about Cindy's current husband, will Cindy talk about how he is different than her ex? If Mellissa talks about her husband instead, will Cindy ask about others before him and will that lead to talking more about her fling. Mellissa, with a heavy feeling in her stomach, dreads the thought of talking about either of those now and bites the tip of her tongue in anxiety.

Cindy looks over at her with a question on her face.

"Sorry I'm quiet. The winding on the road can make me nauseous sometimes." They park the car at a restaurant called the Bubble Room. Looking to break the dull silence, Mellissa asks, "What is the Bubble Room?"

"It's a restaurant. The food is good, but that's not the most common reason why people go there. They have some of the best cakes in Florida. My favorite is the orange cake. It's made with fresh Florida oranges. My husband's favorite is the red velvet cake. Since he's from Nashville too, it's comfort food for him."

"Wow! It is hot today," Mellissa says. It was 2 pm. "This is like hot yoga."

"The walk in the heat will help to loosen your muscles," Cindy says as she lays two towels on the sand.

"No yoga mats?"

"Yoga has been around for five thousand years, long before they made yoga mats and props. In fact, yoga originally started outdoors. The original props were trees and blocks of wood."

Mellissa's eyebrows lift. "I was not aware of that. Are you also saying all yoga started as hot yoga?"

"Not so fast. It *is* hot out here today, but yoga didn't start in Florida. It started in India, which has many different landscapes and climates. There are also many different types of yoga. Most basic gym yoga classes are yoga fit classes. When you talk about hot yoga, the temperature can be up to 110 degrees. Many people like that because they use select postures and they are done over and over again. The repetitions of the postures make it easier to learn and the temperature can more easily get the heart rate up. The heat also has therapeutic qualities; it helps you to let go of things."

Mellissa hopes that is what they are going to do today. She definitely feels like she needs to let some things go.

"My yoga practice is more Iyengar philosophy. I focus on alignment and body balance. We breathe into a pose and hold onto it longer."

Mellissa's attention begins to fade since she thought the hot yoga sounded good.

"Iyengar yoga aims to unite the body, mind and spirit for well-being. It's a powerful tool used to relieve the stresses of modern day life."

Mellissa's attention comes back.

Cindy begins instruction. "Let's begin our poses, our asanas." They start with a couple rounds of sun salutations.

"Nice. Sun salutations in the sun." Mellissa remarks.

"Let's transition to warrior one pose. Put your right foot up and left leg back."

Mellissa mirrors as she connects with the sky. She feels a mixed sense of invigoration and calmness after the deep breaths.

"We will now move to warrior two." The girls go through a series of movements, transitions.

Mellissa feels her leg muscles lengthen with her front knee bent. Her head is turned facing the ocean. She has her arms out like a child pretending to be an airplane, her hands are out, palms up and she feels the warmth of the sun. Normally, when Mellissa does yoga fit at her gym there is calming meditation music in the background. This time, Mellissa hears the crashing of the ocean, birds diving for fish and the rustling of the wind moving through the palm trees.

"We will now move to warrior three. This is a posture of

balancing, just as our life needs to have balance. Your body will be a pendulum. Balance and bring your arms in front of you as if the palms of your hand are holding an inflatable beach ball, send your left leg rising back. Now we will repeat that with the other side of our body," Cindy says as she flows from one pose to the next.

Mellissa goes along with the flow of poses. "Yes, I want both sides of my body to be able to get that nice stretch."

"It is more than that," comments Cindy. "The Indian philosophy in yoga is that the left body is calming and the right body is energizing. We have to have a daily balance. However, not every day is the same. When I wake in the morning, I don't just pop up. I wake up and roll to my side. I think to myself, is this a day where I need to train clients and need energy which requires more of my right body or is this a weekend where I am going to lounge with my husband and start the day by focusing on the calming or left side of my body?"

"The mind influences the body and the body influences the mind," Mellissa quotes Cindy.

"And you feel the way you think," Cindy adds.

The women go through several other poses. Mellissa likes the soft feeling of sand under her towel rather than the yoga mat. Though she is relaxed through the poses, between them she gets intruding thoughts about Cindy. She keeps trying to block out the fact she knows her ex-fiancé. *Cindy is happily married now. Why would Cindy want to know about an exflame that she has moved on from? Why would I keep something from Cindy of this importance? Is it important at all?*

"Mellissa, you seem distracted. You haven't given me much more than one-word responses all day. What's on your mind?"

"Oh, nothing. I mean I have a lot on my mind. Actually, I have a lot of nothing on my mind."

"Mellissa, that is completely normal."

Mellissa gives Cindy a surprised look. "What's normal?"

"The messages in your head. We can have thousands of

messages come through our head. Then we think about our past experiences. We think about tasks and deadlines. It turns into stories about our future based on things that have happened in the past. It is normal. It can be overwhelming."

"It makes me anxious. Then I can feel my heart racing and my mind wanders. How can I keep my mind from wandering? By the way, what time is it? I left my watch in the hotel."

"Anytime you look down at your watch, the time is now," Cindy replies with a calming smile. "Let's try something. Let's get in the shade of the tree, sit and take a deep breath."

They head to the shade of the trees. The sound of the shore is faint and muffled. Cindy turns to Mellissa. "Put one hand on your chest like the Pledge of Allegiance and another on your abdomen between your navel and your rib cage. Breathe normally. Think about which hand you feel moving more."

Mellissa does as instructed and takes a couple of normal breaths. Mellissa sucks in her stomach to keep it from sticking out. Mellissa feels her hand on her chest move slightly and out of the corner of her eye, she sees a bit of her elbow against the horizon.

"Now for thirty seconds, Mellissa, take deep breaths. Each time you breathe out make the exhalation longer than the breathing in. Extend your diaphragm and take a breath to the point where you feel your hand on your abdomen move."

Mellissa feels a calming sensation.

"Each time you exhale, your heart rate slows a bit and your blood pressure relaxes. And that is not yoga but our body physiology. Diaphragmatic breathing relaxes the heart. Relaxing the heart relaxes the mind."

"The mind influences the body and the body influences the mind." Mellissa smiles. She feels more relaxed, but also has a different sensation, almost like a mild euphoria. Maybe it's the sun.

"The deep breath will actually hinge your ribs open and increase your body's oxygen level. You can get ten times the amount in a normal breath. When you move your ribcage and diaphragm, it also moves your belly. Did you know that the majority of your body's serotonin is stored in your gut?"

"What does that have to do with anything? What is serotonin?"

"Serotonin is part of your brain chemistry. It is important for influencing mood. Antidepressants commonly increase our brain levels of serotonin. It helps in treatment of depression and anxiety."

"But if it's in your gut, how does it go to your brain?"

"How does an antidepressant that you swallow go to your brain?"

"Good point. Can I do this anytime? I mean it's not really that practical."

"Why? 'Cause you're a lady and have to hold your belly in?"

Mellissa is unsure if that was a rhetorical question or if Cindy really wants a response.

"I think it's very practical to take thirty seconds and deep-breath as opposed to letting your mind continue to run down a winding road that makes you nauseous with anxiety."

Mellissa doesn't try to block out her thoughts but instead focuses on her breathing.

"Mellissa, when you thought you saw an alligator you looked anxious and you seemed to have grabbed your heart."

"Yes. My heart was pounding."

"And what did that do to your mind?"

"My mind was alert; it scanned everything until I realized it was just a log. That was a relief."

"What do you think your heart and mind do when you're anxious that you're not asleep?"

Mellissa exhales slowly and nods. The point was well taken.

"Let's head back now so we can get you to your session with Lawrence. Namaste," Cindy says. "I bow to you and the divine light and universe that reside within you. We are one."

Paradise Sleep Pearls: Chronic illnesses such as insomnia are influenced by stress. Some have estimated 70% of chronic illnesses are stress related. Relaxation techniques and meditative practice such as body scan, yoga, mindfulness or even sitting meditation have been shown to reduce stress in the forms of anxiety, anger and worry.

Burdick, D. Mindfulness Skills Workbook for Clinicians and Clients. 111 Activities, Worksheets, Techniques & Tools. 2013 Premier Publishing and Media. CMI Education Institute Inc. Eau Claire, WI

Ride Back

On the drive back, they leave the windows up and the air-conditioning on. It seems to be taking longer to get back than it did to get there. Mellissa's mind is fatigued and her eyelids grow heavy. She fights off little sleep episodes.

"I see you are tired. I guess I've done my job once again."

"The sun has zapped the life out me."

"No, Mellissa. Actually, the sun gives us energy. In places with long winters and less sunlight, people actually get fatigued or get seasonal affective depression."

"Then why am I so tired? Why am I always so tired after a day at the beach?"

"It's the drop in your body temperature that makes you tired. That's why a warm bath at night before bed actually helps people sleep. After they get out of the warm bath their body temperature drops and that causes them to be sleepy."

Mellissa looks at Cindy, half-confused. "But I swear the sun makes me tired."

Cindy adjusts the seatbelt across her chest. "You asked why someone is tired after the beach. Let's use today for an example. When you go to the beach, you have been in the sun all day. The heat has been increasing your core body temperature. We also did some physical activity on the beach, increasing your body temperature. You were awake and alert the entire time out there."

Mellissa feeling drowsy nods her head in affirmation.

"The first thing we did when we left was rinse off the sand.

The water actually absorbed some of our body heat. That's actually why people sweat; it helps keep their body from overheating. Next, we came into an air-conditioned space. Then we had a cool drink. And now, we are back in the air conditioning of the car. You are even using your sweatshirt as a blanket because you feel kind of cool from your body temperature dropping. It is the big change in climate that decreased our body temperature and that is what makes us tired."

"So if I can't sleep at night, should I just make myself cold?"

"No. It is the drop from a higher temperature to a cooler body temperature that makes you tired. If your body temperature is normal and you cool yourself, that may make you uncomfortable and will wake you. Your body temperature is lowest in the morning. Many people wake up cold and shivering. So at night, you need to be comfortable so you want to cool down, but not make yourself cold."

Mellissa realizes on early fall days her husband wakes up before she does and turns the heater on. Keeping the temperature steady helps her sleep in a little longer. However, on days he works, the heater isn't turned on and she wakes up earlier, shivering with cold hands and feet from the Nashville autumn chill.

"So a warm bath at night initially increases my body temperature. I feel cold coming out of the shower because the water is absorbing the heat. By the time I have my sleepwear on, I have had a drop in body temperature. That is what makes me sleepy. And my sleepwear keeps me at a comfortable body temperature. It has nothing to do with the lavender bath salts?"

"They work together. The warm bath does loosen your muscles some; it is hard to relax with tense muscles. Where the lavender bath salts come in is association. Your mind learns to associate it with the comfort, relaxed muscles and sleepiness that you get after the warm bath. And when you are in bed, you can still smell the lavender. It reminds you that you are relaxed and you allow yourself to reach a peaceful night sleep."

"Let me guess, the trip out here wasn't so much about the yoga or Captiva for that matter. We took this long trip with the windows down to start feeling the Florida heat. Then we increased our body temperature. And this long ride—which I notice you are driving slower—in this air-conditioned car was to teach me firsthand about drops in core body temperature?"

"Busted! However, with each lesson you get, you are making memories and absorbing visual pictures of our beach paradise. Guided imagery is one of many behavioral sleep techniques. So is relaxation training, and that is part of what we have been doing the past two days on the beach."

"I get it. Insomnia is a beach. These concepts are not unique to sleep only. It's a 24-hour process."

Cindy laughs.

Paradise Sleep Pearls: Relaxing the brain.

The left hemisphere of your brain is your language area; it is logical and likes words. It can be a source of racing thoughts.

The right hemisphere of your brain is creative and imaginative. It also has visual spatial functions and awareness of the body.

When you stimulate the right hemisphere with imagery, the verbal centers of the left hemisphere are effectively shushed. Other methods such as body scan and progressive muscle relaxation can help suppress left brain verbal chatter.

The nerve from your nose is called the olfactory nerve and it has a connection to deep areas of your brain, including the limbic system. The limbic system influences emotion. Just as the scent of warm cookies may be comforting, scents such as lavender or sandalwood may be relaxing.

Siegel, D. Mindsight: The New Science of Personal Transformation. Random House 2010.
Culbert, T. Kajander, R. Be The Boss of Your Sleep: Self-Care for Kids. Free Spirit Publishing Inc. Minneapolis, MN. 2007

Sleep Retreat Session #3: Stimulus Control

"So what do you associate with a good night's rest?"

Mellissa thinks of lavender bath salts, warm baths and traveling. "What do you mean? I really never sleep well. I just can't."

"Never? I thought you were sleeping great here?"

"Never at home. Sanibel and the beach are relaxing. Here isn't the problem. Home is the problem. I never sleep well at home. And I can't just pack my bags and move here like Cindy did."

"Didn't you mention in your survey that you commonly hit snooze on the alarm clock? Wouldn't that mean you were asleep and you are trying to get back to that state?"

"I don't have a problem sleeping so much when I travel and stay at hotels. I can't spend my life traveling. I have to go home."

"So I ask again, you never sleep well? Mellissa, there are things that we can learn to associate with getting to sleep. Have you ever heard of Pavlov's dog?"

"Is this about your corgi again?"

"No. In the 1890, Ivan Pavlov was studying feeding functions in dogs. For part of his research, he needed to isolate saliva from dogs. However, a psychological finding resulted. Noticing that the dogs would begin to salivate before eating, he conducted an experiment where he would ring a bell prior to dinner. Then, there were times when he would ring the bell and not present food to the dogs, yet they still salivated. The dogs had learned to associate the sound of the bell with food."

"Makes sense. Then what? Did the dogs eat too much and fall asleep?"

"That's not the point. There are environmental and behavioral cues that people can learn to associate positively with sleep and rest or negatively with frustration and insomnia. Currently it seems that the site of your bed rings your insomnia bell."

"I still don't understand the point you are trying to make."

"Most people, when they go to a hotel, sleep great. You walk into the room, the bed is made and the room is clean. You are away and associate the time with rest and relaxation. You don't have to pay the electric bill so you crank up the air conditioner and then you curl up in the bed and relax until you fall asleep."

"Makes sense. I do sleep great in hotels and I guess there is a reason why hotel signs have a bed with a person sleeping. But it seems like I don't rest on my last night as I do the first couple nights."

"Sometimes people don't sleep well on their last day. Over the course of a few days, there are some changes. You may be watching television in bed and eating take-out or room service in bed. You are planning daytime activities in bed. People may be in and out of the room. You have your suitcase open, a pile of laundry on the floor and things in your pocket/purse may be on the stands. The bed may not be made because you napped. The room has a cluttered feel to it. What happens is this: when you arrived at that hotel room, you associated it with rest; however, you did so many daytime activities in the room that you lost the association with sleep. It was replaced with all the things you did while awake. Your mind is not able to shut off from the daytime activities."

"I guess I see what you are saying. When I travel I never bring work to bed, instead I go to the business center and I wear a business suit. However, at home I often take my laptop in bed to get work done when I can't sleep. It's a ritual. First I post on Facebook that I can't sleep, then I work the night away."

"When you do daytime things in bed, the bed does not become a place of sleep, but rather an extension of daytime activities. You can't shut your mind off from the associations. And it doesn't help when someone posts on Facebook that they can't sleep. And then they keep checking it to see who else is up. It alerts your mind."

"Wow! I can't count how many times I couldn't sleep in bed so I went to the couch, and next thing I know, my husband is waking me in the morning."

"There is nothing mystical about the couch. What happens is you associate the couch with rest as you may with a nap. But there are negative associations with the bed; thoughts of *I cannot sleep*. This is psychophysiological insomnia."

"That's funny because sometimes I will fall asleep watching a movie on the couch but when my husband wakes me up to go to bed, then I can't sleep. I have always blamed it on his snoring."

"Now for couples, the marital bed is also a place for intimacy, if you enjoy it. If you don't enjoy it, then negative associations will be made. But Mellissa, not to harbor on things you didn't want to talk about but the fling you had...it was in bed, middle of day, then you would get up and go back to work, but have a cigarette first. It almost sounds as if sex energizes you."

"I never thought of it that way. I guess that's why my husband and I have sex more frequently in the morning."

"All that seems pretty wake-promoting. Normally, we say the bed is for sleep or sex only. But I think we say that because Americans are not creative enough to have sex in other places."

"Oh, my God! The other night we were watching a movie and we ended up having sex on the couch. I don't remember the end of the movie. I just remember my husband waking me saying it's time to go to bed. I was asleep, but once he woke me, I couldn't sleep the rest of the night. It's like my bed is a waterbed filled with caffeine."

"Seems like if your bed is caffeine, then your couch is a

fluffy cloud of melatonin and we need to reverse these associa-tions. You know what you really need, Mellissa?"

"Lululemon?"

"Exactly!"

"I was kidding."

"I'm not. You need to go shopping."

"This is the first thing you have ever said that I actually like. But I don't get it."

"The way your room is set up, your sheets, your sleepwear, your curtains, none of it is working for you now. If there were ever a time completely to rearrange your room and redecorate, that time is now. Another option is to just buy a new house, but that would be irrational."

"But I don't sleep in pajamas. I like to get up and run so I sleep in my running sweater."

"Mellissa, you said you fell asleep after sex on the couch the other day. Did you have your running gear on?"

"No. I had a slip on."

"Sounds like when you are dressed at night to get ready for your morning, you have your mind on being awake at a time when you are trying to go to sleep."

"Hmm…I hadn't thought about it that way."

"Yeah, you need to go shopping. I advise you to get a set of pajamas. Do not use old clothes or sweats. Turn over a new leaf. The process of putting on the sleepwear is a transition that marks our association with a sleep ritual. Very important! If the pajamas are comfortable, do not wear them all day when you are home or the association with sleep transition may be lost."

"That is exactly what I'll do."

"I would advise sleepwear you use only for sleep and as-sociate with sleep. Take my wife for example, it doesn't matter the brand, she specifically looks for pajamas with clouds, birds flying, anything that she could associate with the act of flying."

Mellissa cocks her head and squints. *Strange, one only sees clouds and birds flying in the daytime. What does that have to do with sleep?*

Lawrence continues, "My wife loves to read, especially memoirs and people's life stories. She came across a book written by Julie Flygare. J-Fly found out she had narcolepsy while in law school. She had sleepiness and cataplexy. Cataplexy is difficult to explain, but just to simplify it—it's like passing out during an emotional episode. The cataplexy and sleepiness accumulate. It is almost as if the world is her pillow. She has the opposite problem you have. Julie fights to keep her eyes open and stay awake. One thing both of you have in common is that her doctor also suggested her symptoms could be psychologically related. She wrote a great book. She said when she finished it, she wanted to raise her hands and float. So my wife associates anything flying with sleep—not just because Julie Flygare has narcolepsy but because at the end of the day we all dream to be someone special and J-Fly is now living her dream."

Mellissa smiles. "That is inspirational." She then briefly thinks about her niece Samantha. *I'll have to tell Rick about this.* "What about sounds? Should I listen to music if I can't sleep?"

"Do you listen to music in the daytime? In your car while you are trying to stay alert? Do you go out dancing to music and try to stay up? If so, those are going to bring daytime wake promoting thoughts. Sleep-specific stimulus is what is needed."

"You know, Rick has a friend from Puerto Rico. He always talks about how great he sleeps in Puerto Rico when he goes back to visit his family. On the island, there is a frog called *el coqui*. It makes a sweet chirp at night only. You will never hear it in the daytime, unless there is heavy rain that makes people sleepy. He has a smile on his face every time he talks about it."

"This is where I get back to your worries. People with insomnia are frequently very mentally engaged in worries and environmental factors as they try to sleep. Many people with insomnia feel they are victims of their problem. They feel there is nothing that can be done because they think that everything has already been done. It's important to change this victim attitude by developing coping skills for not being able to get to sleep. The active mind cannot shut off and if you put that active mind on the bed, the bed becomes the Pavlov bell of insomnia."

The day three discussion of stimulus control allows her to see the importance of the day two discussion of sleep restriction. Likewise, the day two lesson of sleep restriction helps reduce the day one lesson of psychophysiological insomnia. She realizes she is capable of sleeping and sleeps great in her resorts. "So shopping is the plan? Shopping therapy for sleep to go along with the sleep diet."

"This concept is not unique to sleep. These concepts are called stimulus control. Stimulus control has been used in weight loss by eating when only certain cues are present as opposed to compulsive eating. The president of a weight management company actually helped to develop stimulus control. Again, this further supports my theory that sleep should be approached like weight management."

Paradise Sleep Pearls: Narcolepsy is a disorder of sleepiness, but it is more than that. It is also a problem with regulation of REM sleep. Essentially, REM phenomena occur in the daytime. The most common symptoms are sleepiness, cataplexy, sleep paralysis and hallucinations.

Cataplexy is a loss of muscle tone, a weakness, which occurs most commonly provoked by emotion (such as laughter). Remember, in REM our muscle tone is lower to protect ourselves from acting out our dreams.

In sleep paralysis, one is awake, they know they are awake, but they cannot move and people complain of feeling paralyzed. Once again, it is REM low muscle tone intrusion.

The hallucinations that occur are generally vivid dream like images. Most typically, they occur upon sleep-wake transition.

The average age of onset Narcolepsy symptoms are 15-19 years of age, though it is also common to have symptoms earlier at 10-14 years of age. On average, it takes over seven years from onset of symptoms until a diagnosis is established.

Insomnia is actually another common symptom of Narco-lepsy. It sounds paradoxical that a disorder of sleepiness is associated with insomnia. However just as REM intrusion can occur into wake, wake intrusion can occur into sleep.

Kryger, MH. Principles and Practice of Sleep Medicine: Fifth edition. 2011 Elsevier. Palo Alto, CA

Getting Ready

Mellissa heads back to the hotel to meet Cindy for shopping therapy. She believes stimulus control will be her favorite lesson yet.

She passes the bar and sees Palo again.

Mellissa walks up to Palo. "Are you still going to wait 'till day six of my five night sleep retreat to tell my how you ended up here in Florida?"

"OK. You want to hear the truth?"

"Yes." Mellissa leans forward.

"My father is filthy rich and I don't need to work another day in my life." Palo smiles.

"Ha! You're the prince of Naples, Italy. Coming to America! Let me guess, in search of a bride?"

"I told you, you would not believe me."

"Come on Palo, tell me the truth."

"I did. That is the short version. Maybe on the sixth day, if you have an open mind, I will finish."

Mellissa smiles and walks away. *There is something he is not revealing.*

Paradise Sleep Pearls: Stimulus control for sleep is designed to strengthen the bed as a cue for sleep. Concurrently, it is also designed to reduce bed activities that are not consistent with sleep. The components of this technique include, use the bed for sleep and sex only, go to bed only when sleepy and get out of bed if you are unable to fall asleep. Clock watching is highly discouraged.

Bootzin, R. Behavioral Sleep Medicine Series: Stimulus Control Webinar. American Academy of Sleep Medicine. 2009, March.

Waterside Weasel

The Waterside Shops are outdoors, with white stone everywhere. The outdoor shops are clean and the bright sun seems to radiate between the white stone and the steel rails surrounding the water fountains found on every side of the plaza.

Mellissa looks forward to arranging her room and mind to allow herself to experience a peaceful and restful sleep. She also realizes she has been hard on herself. The more sleepless she has been, the harder she has been on herself. On a clear day, after a few nights of good rest, she is able to better identify her own irrational thoughts.

A store catches her eye. Designer children's clothes hang in the window. She approaches. Stylish diaper bags and heavenly baby blankets start a mental list of things she would like to buy once she gets pregnant. Motivated to keep trying, whether through better sleep, fertility drugs or in vitro procedure, she knows a spark of desire burns within.

They shopped for several hours. The hot Florida day brings a buildup of clouds. The clouds shade the bright sun. A monsoon whooshes down. They didn't bring umbrellas, but it doesn't matter as it lasts only 20 minutes. Now the earth feels cooled by 10 degrees. An ensuing breeze seems to drop the temperature another 5 degrees, just enough to bring a smile. Dusk approaches and a few crickets and cicadas start a light warm up to their upcoming orchestra.

Mellissa has been rather quiet while thinking about all the things she wants to buy. She hasn't opened up to Cindy much. But now, after a day of shopping, Mellissa feels she can let her guard down.

Just then, as if she can read Mellissa's thoughts, Cindy turns to her and asks, "So Mellissa, when do you think you started to have insomnia?"

"I thought about that today when Lawrence was talking about stimulus control. But I know it was in grad school."

"I can understand the stress of grad school."

"Not so much the stress. I had an affair with a man in grad school. It was during my internship. We worked great together and I found him attractive. He told me he was divorced, but in the end, I don't know if he ever was since he ended up with his wife again. He played with my emotions. Even after it was over, there were times that I would stay awake thinking about him. I would look at my phone, waiting for him to call. Now, as a married woman, I feel guilty as if I betrayed my own gender with those thoughts. Maybe I'm over reacting, but that's how I feel."

"You can't blame yourself for having been manipulated. I would be devastated if that happened to me as well. And I couldn't even imagine what it would be like to be on the other side. To be the one that was cheated on. I can hold a grudge. Hell knows no wrath like my grudges."

"I don't know what I was thinking. He was a decade older than I was."

Cindy shakes her head. "I literally don't know what I would do or say to a girl a decade younger than me if she were having an affair with my husband. We don't live in a time of concubines and courtesans. I could see myself losing cool and smacking her."

"Even worse, I am realizing that it was invigorating. He actually introduced me to smoking after sex. Come to find out on this trip that nicotine interferes with sleep."

"It's a bad habit but doesn't make you a bad person. My husband used to smoke when I first met him."

"I didn't want to talk about it. Not even to you at first. It would bring back too many old thoughts. But I appreciate what you did for me at the yoga session with helping me understand that these racing thoughts are normal. And I appreciate the deep breathing techniques."

"If you find your mind drifting back to the quickies you had in grad school, you can use it."

"I have to say one thing…it…" Suddenly, Mellissa stops short as she hears an older man singing a song she remembers.

"The weasel, the weasel. Pop! Pop! Goes the weasel, the weasel. Pop goes the weasel 'cause the weasel goes pop!"

It's a father singing trying to embarrass his teenage daughter around her boyfriend. He sings the old 1990's rap song. Mellissa drops her purse, puts her hand over her heart and feels it beating against her chest.

"You OK, Mellissa?" Cindy peers into her face, concern in her eyes.

"I'm sorry. That startled me."

"I guess we all have memories of our fathers embarrassing us!"

"No, that's not it. It reminded me of something that happened in high school."

"What?"

"When I was in high school, I had a history teacher who would always give us pop quizzes. 'The Weasel' is what he called it. The Weasel was Mr. Carney's friend and he had a strong stench. However, only Mr. Carney could smell him. The Weasel was not into studying and tests so every now and then, while Mr. Carney was teaching, mid-sentence he would sniff and start singing that song. Mr. Carney would give the class a pop quiz to get rid of The Weasel. That song became annoying to everyone, especially me since I was frequently up late on at night and could not study regularly. I was more of a crammer. I still dread the sound of that song."

"Is that why you looked so uncomfortable?"

"No. The last time I heard that song, I was with the guy from my internship. We had just eaten lunch at the mall and we decided to go back to my place, but on the way, we passed a lingerie shop. I was looking at a French Maid slip, a little delight I had picked up in a summer I spent in Paris. I had just asked him if he liked it. Suddenly, the cashier's phone went off and 'The Weasel' was the ringtone. I immediately dropped the French Maid slip to the floor. He looked at it and said, 'It looks great on the floor.'"

"What guy doesn't like a French Maid slip?" She pauses. "I guess we know more about each other than we thought we would." Cindy laughs.

Mellissa thinks about telling Cindy about her ex. She is uneasy however about bringing up the past. Mellissa decides to practice the lesson Cindy taught her. Pushing the thought out of her mind, she focuses on her surroundings. "Let's get some ice cream. My treat. I'll let you burn the calories off of me later."

"I'll hold you to that promise."

They walk into the ice cream shop. The cashier says, "Welcome. We have a special today. It's a walnut sundae, with chocolate ice cream, whipped cream, hot fudge, a cherry and walnuts sprinkled on top."

"I love walnuts!" Cindy says in a high-pitched screech. Her face slightly flushed. She springs to her toes like a ballerina and giggles.

Mellissa drops her purse. *Could it be?*

"You OK? Another bad thought of high school pop quizzes?"

"This is too much!" Mellissa says.

"I agree. Too rich for me now. Hearing the walnut special actually reminds me that my husband and I are going out to dinner tonight. Why don't you join us? Guy won't mind."

Guy won't mind! Mellissa did the same ballerina prance when she saw walnut cupcakes when in her internship romance. Guy was his name. About 10 years ago, Cindy lived in Nashville before she married and moved. Her husband used to smoke. Guy was the one who introduced her to cigarettes after sex about 10 years ago. He was married, said he was getting divorced. *Hell knows no wrath like my grudges!* Mellissa grabs her chest as she feels her heart flutter.

Guy won't mind! Hell knows no wrath like my grudges!
Guy won't mind! Hell knows no wrath like my grudges!

"I'm sorry, Cindy. I have a migraine coming on. I need to go back to the hotel."

Paradise Sleep Pearls: Anxiety causes a stress state. Cortisol is released by the adrenal glands during the stress response. Cortisol then stimulates the amygdala (an area associated with panic). Anxiety makes it difficult to bring attention to our inward thoughts.

This biological stress response stimulates our Fight/Flight sympathetic nervous system brain-heart (our mind-body) response. Repeated sympathetic nervous system activity makes the amygdala more reactive to apparent threats, which in turn increases stress hormone activation. It's a feedback loop as such activation further sensitizes the amygdala. This may trigger panic attacks and even further anxiety based on specific situations.

1. Hanson, R. Buddha's Brain. The Practical Neuroscience of Happiness, Love, and Wisdom. New Harbinger Publications. 2009. Oakland, CA
2. Porges, SW. The Polyvagal Theory. Neuropsychological Foundations of Emotions, Attachment, Communication, Self-Regulation. W. W. Norton and Company, Inc. 2011 New York

Monthly Friend

Cindy insists on driving her back, but Mellissa needs instant separation. No sooner, a taxi pulls up. Mellissa jumps in and heads to the hotel.

When she gets to the carpet in the lobby, she takes her heels off and puts them in her shopping bags. She sees Palo from afar. She shifts her shopping bags to her left hand and covers her forehead, right thumb to fingertip on her temples. Looking down, massaging her temples, she glides through the lobby towards the elevators.

Palo calls out, "Are you OK, Mellissa? You look like you saw a ghost."

"Sorry, Palo, I am just not feeling well." She picks up the pace and scurries the path to her room.

She drops the key card twice trying to unlock the door before she gets it on the third try. She opens the door just enough to squeeze in and slams the door shut. She leans up against the door, standing there for a while in shock. Her legs and feet feel odd. She slides down to a sitting position. She dismisses it, gets up and walks around a little bit in her room. The feeling in her feet relieves just enough for her to lie down on top of her bed.

Her monthly friend and it is not her menstrual cycle, itches, burns and leaves her with an uncontrollable urge to move her legs. She can't predict when it is going to come, Restless Legs Syndrome or RLS. The longer she holds her toes still, the more the urge to move them doubles and the pain quadruples. Notable to resist the urge to scrunch her toes together, a terrible sensation like two white foam coolers screeching as they rub together hits her.

What exactly are the odds her RLS would kick in on the same day she learns Cindy was a walnut-loving, grudge-holding, spouse of a man Mellissa had an affair with?

Guy won't mind! Hell knows no wrath like my grudges!
Guy won't mind! Hell knows no wrath like my grudges!
Guy won't mind! Hell knows no wrath like my grudges!
Walnuts! Walnuts! Walnuts!

"Stop!" Mellissa yells to the empty room. She places her head between her knees and sees her toes. The burning in her toes is too much so she wiggles them, but this provokes an inner screech. Mellissa lets go of her ears and grabs her feet, massaging her toes and the skin webbing between. The words come back.

Guy won't mind! Hell knows no wrath like my grudges!
Guy won't mind! Hell knows no wrath like my grudges!
Guy won't mind! Hell knows no wrath like my grudges!
Walnuts! Walnuts! Walnuts!

I can't live this way! I have to get some sleep tonight. Mellissa takes an over-the-counter sleep aid in her toiletry bag. She walks around the room, pacing back and forth from the bed to the bathroom, to the window, to the door, back to the bed and back and forth again. And again. And again.

She lies back down and takes some deep breaths. She feels crawling on her legs and jumps out of the bed and yells, "What the heck, ants in the bed!"

She smacks her legs trying to brush the ants off but there are no ants. She uncovers the sheets and looks at the bed. She can hear her nephews singing, "The ants are marching one by one. Hurrah! Hurrah!" The over-the-counter sleep aid kicks in. A mental fog starts to roll in.

Mellissa is at a breaking point. She grabs her suitcase and starts to pack. First thing when she wakes up, she is heading out of here. Her phone starts to ring. "Mom!"

"Mel, my honey bee," her mother responds.

"I am so glad to hear your voice, Mom. I need your help."

"Are you OK? What's the matter, dear? You sound upset."

"Where do I start? I'm in Florida and Rick is in Nashville. I'm here because I can't sleep or get pregnant. So I am seeing a psychologist, not a psychiatrist. We really haven't talked too much about sleep. Somehow, everything comes back to sex. I see this girl Cindy every day and every day she exhausts me. I slept with her husband, but I didn't mean to. Now my monthly friend is here. I need your help!"

"What? I'm glad you have a psychiatrist there 'cause you're out of your mind!"

"No, Mom, it's not like that. He is a psychologist not a psychiatrist."

"Honey, you need to slow down. First, what are you doing in Florida without your husband?"

"OK. You know I've been trying to get pregnant. And you know I have had insomnia for some time now. Well, I saw a fertility specialist and it turns out that he believes my infertility is related to poor sleep. So I found this sleep retreat in Florida. It's five days long and I only have two days left."

"Goodness, you had to go to Florida to get Xanax?"

"No, Mom. I'm not supposed to take any meds because I'm trying to get pregnant. Anyhow, we have daily sessions for behavioral sleep therapy. There is a personal trainer and day coach here. Her name is Cindy. Every day we do some type of physical activity, which we so far either do at the crack of dawn or in the Florida heat."

"I can see how that is exhausting. How do you have the energy to sleep with her husband? And what on earth possessed you to sleep with him and cheat on your husband?"

"No, Mom. I never told you this, but when I was in grad school, I had a fling with someone."

"That is not how I raised my daughter!"

"Let me explain. We worked well together during my internship. He was funny and charming, and he told me he was divorced."

"Oh, I failed you as a mother."

"No, Mom. I actually now, more than ever, understand how hard you had to work as a woman in a man's world to achieve everything you did. Anyway, his name was Guy and he liked walnuts. It turns out that Cindy is married to a man named Guy who likes walnuts."

"Mellissa, I remember that name and I remember him as a womanizer."

"You remember this so suddenly?"

"Guy came to the restaurant all the time. He mostly came in with his wife. She had short blonde hair. She was really into fitness and the sweetest thing. She loved to look at her diamond ring. It had rubies on each side of it, her birthstone. It broke my heart to see that sweet thing knowing her husband was with a different girl all the time. So one day, I pulled Cindy aside and told her. I'll never forget that moment!"

"Why? Because she was devastated?"

"No because she slapped me. I mean, yes, she looked deflated"

"She slapped you?"

"She was going to get a divorce. But it looks like they worked through their problems, isn't that sweet?"

"No, Mom. It's not sweet. Cindy thinks they worked through their problems, but that is the same exact time I was with him. I can't tell her I slept with him! I have to get out of here. I'm taking the first plane back to Nashville tomorrow."

"You can't do that to yourself. You went down there with a purpose and you are more than halfway through. You owe it to yourself to finish. If you can't get pregnant because of poor sleep, wow, it's great if that's something that you can fix. And I have no doubt in my mind that you will be the greatest mother. I feel I was never there for you during those critical years. Why don't you just take a Midol so you will be able to think more rationally?"

"No, Mom, I'm not having my period. It just seems like once a month I get these bouts of restless legs."

"Oh, that's it? Just take a warm bath and massage your legs." Mellissa's mother laughs. "That's what works for me."

Mellissa exhales. "I'm coming with you next year to Central America. I really want to help with your mission."

"Not if you're pregnant, dear. I promise to be around for your kids. It's like a second chance in motherhood."

"I love you, Mom. I have to go. I actually have to unpack my bags now. I'm going to go through with this. You're right. I have to do what is right."

"That's my honey bee. Always be true to yourself. Good night."

Mellissa decides to soak with lavender bath salts. She still feels the burning sensations of RLS. She thinks back to the lesson Cindy gave her about trying to think about something else. She focuses intently on the scent of the lavender. She massages her legs and feet. She pictures herself walking through a grass field, remembering the feeling of grass blades on her bare feet as a child. She allows thoughts to leave, just as quickly as they come. She stays in the bath until the feeling of the pruneyness replaces that of the RLS.

She makes a point not to look at her phone or a clock while she gets ready for bed. Instead, she calls the front desk and asks for a wakeup call. She quickly hangs up before the clerk can tell her how many hours are left until the call. Instead of trying to force her eyes to close, she paradoxically focuses on keeping them open. As she stares at the ceiling fan, her eyelids grow heavier and heavier. She visualizes her eye muscles resting. They feel tighter and tighter, like a rubber band stretching to its max. By focusing on keeping her eyes open, she diverts racing thoughts until she finally falls asleep.

Paradise Sleep Pearls: Paradoxical intent is a behavioral approach to insomnia. Attempting to force oneself to sleep can lead to Psychophysiological Insomnia. With paradoxical intent, instead one remains passively awake without any effort to fall asleep. It is partially designed to reduce the anxiety of not being able to sleep. Commonly one is gradually relieved as they learn to accept quiet wakefulness as an acceptable alternative. This allows one's natural sleep drive to build until the individual is ready for sleep.

Morgenthaler, T. Et al. Practice Parameters for the Psychological and Behavioral Treatment of Insomnia. SLEEP 2006. Volume 29, Issue 11

Sleep Retreat Session #4:
Cognitive Experiment

Mellissa receives her wakeup call the next morning. She's shocked it's waking her up, since she didn't think she would get any sleep. Mellissa didn't think her mind would rest at all last night. She's amazed her new tactics work.

Awake and feeling exhausted, she is overwhelmed by six degrees of separation everyone seems to have linked to her. *It's as if there are only five people in this world and they all moved from Nashville to Sanibel. Weird.*

Mellissa gets up and looks at her phone. She calculates almost five hours of sleep. That disappoints her. She has a cup of coffee in her room but that's not enough to wake her up. She heads to the nearest coffee shop and orders the largest size they have. She doesn't want to be late for the session with Lawrence. She is not sure why the day was switched around, but figures they must have a good reason. She drives faster than she knows she should. She just can't control her impulses in such a sleep-deprived state. Suddenly she sees swirling lights and hears a siren.

"Busted!" Mellissa rolls down her window and before the young officer can even move his lips, she says, "Let me guess, you are going to invite me to the annual Florida State Trooper Ball?"

The young gun reaches his hands to his dark sunglasses and tips them just enough so Mellissa can see his eyes. He furrows his brow and says, "Ma'am, Florida State Troopers don't have balls."

Mellissa looks him in the eye and doesn't flinch, just holds his gaze steadily and allows an odd silence to take course.

The young officer pushes his sunglasses back up and says, "Drive safe today," before walking back to his car.

Mellissa enters the office, feeling like a hot mess. Guilt and remorse are Mellissa's new companions. She knows she needs to talk with Cindy and tell all. It's the right thing to do. But she doesn't want to involve Lawrence in the whole sordid thing so she chooses not to reveal anything that's happening.

"So how many cups of coffee is this for you?" says Lawrence, upon her arrival.

"How do you know I've had more than one? Do you have little cameras following me around?"

"No cameras. I know you've had more than one cup because I listen to you. You told me that you never leave the house without having a cup of coffee. That tells me this is at least your second cup. I also observe you every day. You are usually very fashionable, but today you look like a train wreck with your mismatched clothing and dark bags under your eyes."

"Gee, thanks. Tell me how you really feel."

"You're welcome. Now tell me, what happened last night?"

"I didn't sleep well. I get occasional RLS. I feel like fire ants are on my feet, but that would be better because I could at least brush those off. I ended up taking an over-the-counter sleep aid, but not even that helped."

"You didn't actually take a product with an antihistamine, did you?"

"I needed to be able to sit here and tolerate your sarcasm the next day, so how else was I supposed to get sleep? And why do you hate sleep meds so much?"

"I don't hate sleep meds. The problem is that people become dependent on them when they have never had a proper sleep evaluation. Everybody uses sleep aids from time to time. Sometimes, on a long flight, patience comes nicely with mimosa and a Valium."

Mellissa laughs, thinking of Jez.

"Both alcohol and Valium do make you sleepy, but they also relax your airway. If you snore, that will make your snoring and your sleep worse. I am not anti-medication; I am pro-what-are-you-treating. Your RLS for example. Many common over-the-counter products and other antihistamines will make those symptoms worse. RLS could also be a sign of low iron levels."

"But I don't have anemia. Some meds can make RLS worse? I didn't know that. That actually explains why after taking that it felt like gasoline over fire."

"Half of these over-the-counter products contain some type of antihistamine. And yes, it makes RLS symptoms worse. It's also a very common misconception among doctors that you have to have anemia in order to benefit from iron therapy when RLS symptoms are present. Just because your blood iron levels are normal, doesn't mean that your brain iron or ferritin levels are normal."

"I am going to be a mess today. And you won't let me nap because of your sleep diet. I am going to have to drop out today."

"Why are you going to be a mess today?"

"I need eight to nine hours of sleep to function. If I get any less, the anxiety and fatigue are overwhelming."

"Mellissa, let's talk about core sleep. The other day you asked if REM sleep was your deep sleep. But REM sleep is actually very active brain time. You are consolidating memories in REM, which is why you may have a dream of someone you hadn't seen in about 10 years."

"Oh! That makes sense."

"Your sleep cycles between REM and Non-REM sleep throughout the night—about every 90 minutes or so. Just as a washing machine cycles between rinse and spin, your sleep has cycles as well."

"That explains why I can have more than one dream in a night."

"Yes and REM sleep cycles are actually more prominent

in the second half of sleep. This would also explain why you remember a dream when your alarm goes off."

"Where are you going with this?"

"Deep sleep that occurs in the first half of the night is core sleep. Similar to how a washing machine has a deep soak in the early cycles. Non-REM sleep has different levels and the deepest most refreshing part of the sleep cycles occurs in the first part. Even during many bad nights of sleep, it's very likely that you experience the core sleep that occurs within the first four hours. Getting less than four hours can be dangerous; in fact, it has been shown to cause traffic accidents at the level of drinking-and-driving. But if you get your core sleep you are OK and like we discussed yesterday, we will use that bit of fatigue you have from not sleeping more than a few hours the night before to help get to bed earlier the next day."

The hair on her neck gives an eerie sensation. She reaches back and scratches. "I'll be right back. I need some water." She walks back to the waiting room where there is a water cooler.

She comes back into the room. Lawrence is patiently sitting. Mellissa sits, crosses her legs and decides to continue with the session. "I apologize. Anyway, I'll go to sleep earlier tonight and eventually on a more regular basis. But what am I going to do about today? Daytime? Remember, it's a 24-hour process."

"It's OK, Mellissa. I'll tell you what we will do about today. Why don't we conduct a cognitive behavioral experiment?"

"That's not funny. I am not a lab rat. I'm telling you my fears and just don't need your sarcasm now. Are you going to make me walk through a maze carrying a pillow looking for a bed?"

"A cognitive behavioral experiment is actually a treatment. We are going to play these scenarios in our heads and then you are going to practice this today and report back to me tomorrow. You have nothing to lose if it works. And I actually think you will be able to function today. If it doesn't work, you were going to drop out today anyway."

"Sorry, I'm just not thinking right because I didn't sleep well last night."

"You believe if you don't get eight hours, you won't be able to function. But it's not all or nothing. Mellissa, you have negative thoughts about sleep. This leads to stress. Then, when you don't sleep well, you start monitoring yourself more. You begin noticing every symptom of tiredness or anxiety. The way you cope with this is by drinking more coffee or smoking a cigarette.

"Have you ever felt like you got a poor night's sleep but still got through the day? Have you ever slept great but still felt fatigue at the end of the day? There are multiple factors that play into daytime fatigue and affect how you feel from day to day."

"I see your point. In the past I have indeed kicked butt during meetings and presentations despite not sleeping well."

"So let's talk more about this selective monitoring because it makes you feel unrested. Feeling like it's too hard to concentrate leads to thoughts of hopelessness or panic. By the way, thoughts of panic and fear are incompatible with sleep. Have you ever had a dream that you were walking and missed a step and then jumped and woke up?"

"Yes!" Mellissa laughs. "That happens to everyone."

"True, everyone I have ever asked that question agrees it has happened to them too. However, I have yet to meet someone who says they have finished a dream in which they fall and crack their head."

"OK, I get your point. You can't panic and have anxious thoughts and expect to sleep. It ends up leading back to psychophysiological insomnia."

"Very good! Now, let's talk about daytime thoughts. Mellissa, you predict that after a night of poor sleep, you will feel terrible the next day and there is nothing you can do to help that. But there are things that can be done to generate energy regardless of sleep. Energy-generating thoughts can be a breath of fresh air as can lunch with a friend or taking a walk on a crisp day."

"I don't really feel like doing that when I'm sleep-deprived, though."

"But your lack of sleep last night has created an opportunity." Lawrence goes on, "You monitor yourself all day for fatigue. If you look for trouble, you will find trouble. If you look for signs of fatigue, you will find them even if you become fatigued about looking for fatigue."

"I currently feel I have sore eyes, heavy head and heavy shoulders."

"You are internally focusing and looking for these symptoms."

"It's what I have always done. These are the thoughts that have always come to my mind."

"Let's brainstorm ideas to test."

"When I feel this fatigued, I don't even want to go shopping. The thought of trying on clothes, taking off what I have on, putting something else on and then if it doesn't fit...I generally just like to stay home when I feel this way."

"Sounds like every time you get up the inertia it takes to do so, makes you feel zapped?"

"It takes the life out of me. It's late, I am already fatigued and having to exert my leg and back muscles into a rising position causes additional fogginess in my mind."

"Go shopping today. Go to Coconut Point, the outdoor mall. I want you to walk around for thirty minutes. I want you to monitor every sign of fatigue that you have. Monitor each time your eyes droop. Occasionally sit down and make a mental note of which muscles in your body feel tight. You are going to miss your CrossFit session with Cindy to do this experiment."

Mellissa is quiet. It's sadistic to make her do something she didn't want to do because she feels exhausted. However, what she wants most is to avoid Cindy.

"Then I want you to walk around again for another thirty minutes. I specifically want you to think about something different than how you are feeling.

"Before you leave to do this experiment, there are a few things I would like to mention. I commonly see dysfunctional beliefs about sleep. For example, a belief bad sleep always equals a bad day. Or that sleep is unpredictable or random. These thoughts become anxiety provoking. Eventually, these irrational beliefs become the causes of chronic insomnia instead of just occasional bad nights."

"I believe that the insomnia is out of my control and that there is something inherently wrong with me. I ask myself every night, 'What is wrong with me?'"

"Do you feel these thoughts prior to sleep overwhelming you?"

"When I think of sleeplessness, it stresses me out and I get emotional."

"I would like to discuss the top five myths about sleep and insomnia: One: I need eight hours of sleep to function. Two: Medication is the only solution. Three: A poor night of sleep ruins the whole week. And four: Insomnia is caused by a chemical imbalance that cannot be fixed."

Lawrence pauses and smiles.

"OK, so what's the fifth? And what is so funny?"

"I just thought of a joke. How do you keep an insomniac in suspense?"

"How?"

"I'll tell you tomorrow!"

Paradise Sleep Pearls: Cognitive therapy for insomnia aims to change the negative thoughts about sleep into positive ones. Such negative thoughts are commonly associated with heightened levels of anxiety. The basic elements of cognitive therapy include shifting the patient away from attributions that are inconsistent with good sleep. Also, there is an attempt to control attributing too much to the consequences of a bad night.

Harvey, A. Behavioral Sleep Medicine Series: Cognitive Approaches to Insomnia Treatment – Behavioral Experiments Webinar. American Academy of Sleep Medicine. 2009, April.

Coconut Tired

Mellissa conducts the behavioral experiment. Though she normally doesn't like to shop when she is tired, she is relieved the CrossFit session with Cindy was cancelled. She walks around the outdoor shopping center and monitors every sign of fatigue. She focuses diligently on what she feels when she is tired: her legs; back; shoulders and how her head droops in fatigue.

She follows Lawrence's directions and the next thirty minutes, rather than monitor for signs of fatigue, she thinks about how to get her mind off being tired. She doesn't even look inside the shops. She notices the texture of the coquina shell like area. She looks at the different flowers in the area, the blooming birds of paradise. She notes the architecture has a Latin feel to it. She passes by the middle square, which has a large fountain around it. There are restaurants and people having lunch outside. Mellissa sits down by a bench facing the fountain.

One family has a squirming child. The mother looks frantic. "This place is not child friendly," she grumbles. "And where is our waitress?"

She overhears the husband say, "Why don't you go inside and wash your hands? Maybe our drinks will arrive by then."

The mother goes inside for a moment.

"Excuse me, miss!" He hails the waitress. "Here is a ten-dollar bill. I need a fifty-cent roll of pennies."

"I'm sorry, sir. We don't give change," The young waitress replies.

"Keep the change please. I just want a fifty-cent roll of coins." He hands her the ten-dollar bill, and in less than a minute, the waitress is back with a roll of coins and drinks for the table.

The wife comes back out. The husband says, "See, sometimes we just need a moment." He takes the roll of pennies out of his pocket and gives one to his son. "Go throw this penny in the fountain son. And make a wish."

The son runs towards the fountain. He passes Mellissa. He looks at the fountain and throws the penny in the water. The little boy jumps and claps in happiness. Then he turns around and runs back.

"Dad, can I have another one." The father gives him another penny. "Dad, can I have more than one."

"No. You can only have one at a time," the father replies. As the little boy bolts back to the fountain, the man looks at his wife and says, "I can have him do this up to fifty-times until all our food comes out."

Mellissa laughs. She gets up and continues to walk. The experience made her think about the pleasant parts of being with family—the smiles on her niece and nephew's faces. Time passes, Mellissa doesn't even want to look at her watch as she aimlessly walks.

She realizes she felt exhausted in her first walk but a rush of adrenaline replaces it as she heads to her car. She realizes the more she thought about her exhaustion, the more her body felt those sensations. But when she thought about other things, those sensations went away. She went from feeling fatigued to being full of energy.

Paradise Sleep Pearls: Overcoming Fatigue

Sitting in an erect posture provides internal feedback to the reticular formation–a mesh like network of nerves in the brainstem, which is involved with wakefulness and consciousness—telling it you need to stay vigilant and alert. This is a neurological reason behind a schoolteacher's demand to "sit up straight, class!" As well as the classic meditation instruction to sit upright in a dignified way.

To overcome drowsiness, it sometimes is suggested you literally visualize light. This brightening technique involves a surge of norepinephrine throughout the brain.

Burdick, D. Mindfulness Skills Workbook for Clinicians and Clients. 111 Activities, Worksheets, Techniques & Tools. 2013 Premier Publishing and Media. CMI Education Institute Inc. Eau Claire, WI

Life in the Fast Lane

Dusk comes as Mellissa heads back to the hotel. The sounds of tranquility quickly fade to a large party of girls laughing.

"I hate sex because I always end up missing a pair of socks," one girl says while the group laughs.

Mellissa walks to the outdoor bar. She sees Palo. "What's the commotion about?"

"Hi Mellissa! It's a bridal party. The bridesmaids are getting to know each other. They are playing a game. They all write down why they hate doing laundry. However, when they read the response, they have to replace laundry with, 'I hate sex because...'"

Another girl laughs before she reads, "I hate sex because you constantly need to buy new supplies."

Mellissa sits down. "That's an ice breaker if I ever heard one. Laundry makes my back hurt. I better not say that one out loud."

"What was troubling you yesterday, Mellissa?" Palo asks while mixing a mojito.

Mellissa looks down and exhales. She spent an entire day taking in the peace within paradise; she wasn't ready just yet to approach the storm within it.

"I'm sorry. I could tell it bothers you still." Palo places the mojito on a cocktail napkin in front of her.

"No, I'm sorry Palo. Something I have to deal with. But I talked with my mother last night and she helped me through it."

"It's always good to be able to just pick up the phone and call your mother or father." Palo smiles.

"Well, even that is not that simple. My mother is in and out of the country. She goes to Central America a lot, to places not even on the map."

"Your mother sounds like an adventurer!"

"It's not like that either. She's a missionary. She goes to areas that are the poorest of the poor. She brings food, builds schools and provides hope."

"Wow! Someone just doesn't wake up and do that. What was her inspiration?"

"It's a story."

"I like stories." Palo comes around the bar and sits next to Mellissa.

"My father was a giving man. He would take leftovers to the homeless and would close the restaurant to the public on slow nights, inviting kids and families from single-parent homes to eat for free and enjoy a talent show. His former employees, aspiring artists who had made it big, would come back on those nights to be part of the talent show and teach the kids how to play instruments or carry a note. It provided hope, especially as the children grew towards adolescence. When my father died, our family was of course devastated. However, the outpour of the community and the people he had influenced along the way brought a solace that my mother could have never imagined. Never in their wildest dreams did they think the single parent families they were trying to provide a break from reality to would be the ones to help through our new reality. One of the kids my father helped made it big. He traveled the world, returning to his home in Nashville between trips and visiting the restaurant. Many of these trips were to Central America through a mission, which went to the poorest areas. My mother started going with him on these trips. She now goes a couple times per year for days to weeks at a time. Miracles in action."

"Tragic that your father died."

"It was a head-on collision that occurred in the middle of the night. I was actually waiting for him that night to tuck me into bed. They were able to determine the driver had been driving for over 24-hours straight."

Palo shakes his head. "So the driver of the other car probably fell asleep at the wheel."

At that moment, Mellissa feels the same odd sensation in her neck from this morning's session with Lawrence. Palo tries talking to her, but Mellissa can't make out the words. He sounds as if talking under water. Palo makes a motion to Mellissa, pointing at the party. His body language shows the need to tend to the party. Mellissa shakes her head and heads back to her room.

Paradise Sleep Pearls: There is a higher incidence of automobile accidents with self-reported sleep disorders. Sleep deprivation accounts for more automobile accidents then driving and texting. Some studies have suggested that driving sleepy may be as dangerous as driving intoxicated, and driving while intoxicated and sleepy is even more dangerous. When a car accident results in death, though you can measure a blood alcohol level on the dead body to provide a statistic, postmortem measurements of sleep deprivation cannot be assessed.

1. Pack AI, Pack AM, Rodgman E, Cucchiara A, Dinges DF, Schwab CW. Characteristics of crashes attributed to the driver having fallen asleep. Accid Anal Prev 1995; 27:769-775
2. Knipling RR, Wang JS. Crashes and fatalities related to driver drowsiness /fatigue. Research note. Washington, DC: National Highway Traffic Safety Administration, November; 1994

Bottle Opener

Mellissa gets out of bed a little earlier than usual feeling refreshed. She sees a text from Cindy suggesting they double up today, CrossFit in the morning and later wind surfing after the sleep session. Mellissa's replies with a short: I leave for the airport after the last session today.

On the way to the lobby, Mellissa practices what she plans to tell Cindy as the time has come. "I slept with your husband." *That's not going to work.* "What if she tries to slap me?"

Cindy laughs and asks, "What are you doing?"

Mellissa realizes she made it to the lobby and right to Cindy. "I'm sorry."

"It's OK. We all have odd moments." Cindy smiles.

"No Cindy, honestly, I'm sorry. I have done you wrong in ways you can't imagine and I'm sorry." Mellissa breaks eye contact for just a moment and looks at Cindy's wedding ring. There are rubies on each side of the diamond. "Were you born in July?"

"You're sorry I was born in July? Why are you acting so weird?" Cindy furrows her brow.

"I'm not acting. I am weird. I mean…I feel weird. I mean…"

"What is going on?"

Mellissa takes a deep breath and sits before looking Cindy in the eye. She tries to speak but instead pauses and scoots herself away from Cindy's reach.

Cindy looks confused and curious.

"I know your ex-fiancé in Nashville. He is my doctor. And I remember him from the moment he moved there. I made the connection when you started talking about the behavioral sleep."

"Why didn't you say anything then?"

"I wasn't sure at first, but when you made the paradise in Kauai comment, there was no doubt. I remember he used to talk about his plans to go there with his fiancée, which must have been you."

"So you are his patient?" Cindy's body language is uncomfortable, but she hasn't cocked her arm back—yet.

"Yes, I was his patient," Mellissa says, nodding. "I recently decided to leave the practice, though."

Cindy sighs. "I can understand why it would be odd. It must have been tough on you to hold it in. Oh, well. It's not like you had a relationship with him." After an idle pause, Cindy's ears and neck flush. She looks at Mellissa. "Why would you leave his practice? He worked hard to build it. It cost us our marriage."

"Cindy, I thought you said you guys grew apart? Anyhow, that is not the only thing. I do have to talk to you about a relationship, a fling that I now regret."

Beet red with anger, Cindy yells, "So you did sleep with him! Have you no shame?"

The entire hotel lobby turns to watch them. Palo walks over. He asks, "Signoras, can we calm down and take this outside, please?"

Mellissa feels the wave of embarrassment wash over her as everyone in lobby eyeballs her. She tries to talk. Her jaw and lips move but no words come out. Mellissa feels the pressure of bottled up emotions and embarrassment shaking through her body.

Cindy ignores Palo, leans forward and gives Mellissa a disgusted look. She practically spits, "You know, I feel sorry for your husband. You're no honeybee. You couldn't have been more misnamed."

The pop of a cork sounds in Mellissa's head. The bottled

emotions escape. "I didn't sleep with your ex-fiancé the lousy doctor! But I did sleep with your husband!"

Cindy looks completely dumbfounded. She stands there, motionless like an old Nashville hickory tree. Palo takes a step back and says, "OK, signoras."

"Your husband used to dine at my family's restaurant in Nashville. He brought you there, but he also brought other women there frequently. My mother felt sorry for you and couldn't watch it anymore, so she approached you about it. She really liked you and couldn't stand that a womanizer was deceiving you. Do you remember slapping her?" Mellissa takes a step back.

"These are some tangled webs you are weaving!"

"Wall nuts. I swear I didn't know it was you. It only came to me when we were shopping the other day. When we talked about French Maid outfits. I was sure when you told me your husband's name is Guy."

"Does anyone have a cigarette?" Palo asks.

In a split second, Cindy's beet red anger turned into cherry red pain. "Why would he have done this to me?" She takes a couple of wobbly steps while moving her hands around as if reaching for something in the dark. She passes out and starts to grow pale.

Mellissa approaches Cindy. She clasps Cindy's left hand with her own. She puts her right arm around Cindy's back and guides her to a chair. Mellissa leans in and hugs Cindy. "I said that I felt like I betrayed my own gender. And you've already slapped my mother and yelled at me in a hotel lobby filled with guests. Who are still watching us, might I add."

"I guess we can call it even," Cindy remarks as she starts to cry.

Palo turns to the crowd gathered in the lobby. "The show's over. Let's get on with our lives."

In a perfect world, Guy would have held true to his solemn vows to be Cindy's faithful partner in sickness and health. And, in that same perfect world, a sleep-deprived driver wouldn't have taken away Mellissa's father and she would have been tucked into bed every night as a child.

They sit there quietly for a while until Cindy stops crying. Cindy dabs her eyes with the edge of her shirt and says, "You heard Palo, let's get on with our lives."

Paradise Sleep Pearls: Adjustment insomnia is a short term form of insomnia. The onset of adjustment insomnia generally coincides with something of importance that just occurred in a person's life and is routinely caused by stress, anxiety or some form of depression or worry. It typically lasts anywhere from a few days to a few months at maximum.

As many as 20% of adults deal with acute insomnia at least once each year and over 90% of adults will deal with it at least once in their lives (THE OTHER 10% MAY BE IN DENIAL).

Jacobs GD. Say Good Night to Insomnia, The Six-Week, Drug-Free Program Developed At Harvard Medical School. Henry Holt and Co. Holt Paperbacks September 2009

Sleep Retreat Session #5:
Sleep Hygiene is Crap

Mellissa packs her bags and carry-on into the rental car. She hopes to leave her emotional baggage in the hotel lobby. Mellissa heads to the last session. "Home stretch," she says to herself. She can't wait to get home—but no speeding this time.

Mellissa walks into Paradise Sleep. The door to Lawrence's office is open. Mellissa sits on the old-fashioned psychiatry couch, kicks her shoes off and puts her feet up.

Lawrence walks in and looks up from his iPad. "How did your experiment go?"

"It went well. I didn't want to admit it to you but when I left Coconut Point, I actually felt a lot better. I made it through the day just fine."

"Good. So the joke is on you!"

"I'm sorry. I don't understand."

"I didn't finish my top five insomnia beliefs…drum roll! Number five: They feel they can't manage negative sleep consequences the next day."

Mellissa exhales with a sigh. "Why exactly do you make this a five-night retreat? I mean you could make it a full-day seminar or even do this on the web."

"Commitment and belief. Day one begins before you arrive, the moment the phone is picked up and the commitment is made to come for five days. People talk about change, they talk about losing weight or making New Year's resolutions, but it's the power of commitment that makes the diet and exercise a lifestyle change that will lead to success. The person who hires a personal trainer and a nutritionist is going to be more successful in achieving their New Year's resolution than a person who seeks fat-burning supplements at their local vitamin store. Likewise, the person who believes they can concur sleep and embarks on a six day period of learning is more likely to stay committed six weeks or six years from now. This is actually day six for you, Mellissa."

Mellissa's eyebrows rise. *Palo said he would tell his story on day six. He must have gone through the program himself.*

Lawrence continues, "And those who do not believe they can sleep, they deserve help too. But most commonly the place to start is not with a sleep retreat but rather with automatic negative thoughts; those ANTs can consume one's mind more than any other physical disease ever can."

Mellissa shakes her head. Her mind is clear, her conscience is clear. "I brought the sleep hygiene list you asked for. I still haven't looked at the ten sleep hygiene tips. I don't think I ever would have."

"Concepts are more important than instructions." Lawrence takes the sheet from Mellissa. "I am going to read through your sleep hygiene list and then let's talk about the whys.

> Sleep Hygiene:
> One: Don't nap.
> Two: Go to bed at the same time.
> Three: Do not exercise at night.
> Four: If you cannot sleep, get out of bed and read a boring book.
> Five: Do not watch TV or read in bed.
> Six: Do not go to bed angry.
> Seven: Use the bed for sleep or sex only.
> Eight: Have a comfortable mattress.
> Nine: Do not study or work in bed.
> Ten: Do not drink caffeine at night.

"You know, they have actually done studies where all they do is just give a patient a list of sleep hygiene for insomnia and consistently it has proven to be unhelpful. Oftentimes in trials for treatment of insomnia, the non-treatment group simply gets a sleep hygiene list just like this."

"So sleep hygiene is not important?"

"It's actually very important. Cardinal important. But when I say sleep hygiene is crap, what I am referring to is just giving someone a list without any explanation—that doesn't work. Sleep hygiene needs to be individualized as well as explained. And I don't agree with all of these items on this list at all. Let's go through it together.

"One: Don't nap. Actually, what you want to do is avoid daytime naps lasting two or more hours. It's 3 pm now. If you leave and go eat a burger and fries, will you be hungry for dinner at 6 pm? No. Just as a person has a hunger drive, you also build a sleep drive throughout the day. If you take a long nap, you curb some of that sleep drive and you won't be able to sleep at night. However, a twenty-to-forty-minute nap has been shown to be helpful for alertness.

"Two: Go to bed at the same time. It's more important to be consistent with your wake time. Look, you cannot control if you have to work late. However, when you sleep in late, you aren't going to have that same sleep drive that evening. If you get a little less sleep one night, but wake up at your regular time, then you will get to sleep better the next evening. And in fact, when you do get to sleep you will rebound with more deep sleep."

"Three: Do not exercise at night. I especially don't like this one. I feel that people need to exercise when they can. There's nothing wrong with a walk after dinner. The point is to try and not exercise to the point of sweating within one hour of going to bed. It raises your core body temperature and can make getting to sleep difficult. But if you only have time to exercise at night, you are better off doing that than letting a decade go by and letting your health go. I have never heard anyone say that they haven't exercised in weeks and they feel great.

"Four: If you cannot sleep, get out of bed and read a boring book. Gag me with a bookmark! Seriously, if I am frustrated that I can't sleep, the last thing I want to do is something that I hate doing. Part of the problem with insomnia is that people worry that they can't sleep. So now I have to choose between worrying that I can't sleep or purposely irritating myself? It is more important to do something you enjoy but specifically that you associate with sleep and winding down. It is really important to get out of bed if you cannot sleep. Stay awake in your bed for too long and you will learn to associate your bed with frustrations about not getting to sleep.

"Five: Do not watch TV or read in bed. The emphasis should be on reducing activities that may wake you up before bedtime, such as TV, video games, internet, cleaning, thinking or planning in bed. Why? Because you're using wakeful brain rhythms and thoughts, which will keep you awake. I once went to a seminar given by Michael Perlis. To me, he is the number one insomnia expert. During the seminar, he said that he reads in bed. The crowd went silent and everyone looked at him. Then he explained that he has been working on the same book for over a year. It's not that he doesn't like the book; it's just that it is something that relaxes him and helps him get to sleep. He's even had to start the book over because he forgets parts of it. He has tried to read it during the daytime to experiment, and even then he fell asleep to it."

Mellissa can relate. "Wow! That's why I fall asleep when I read my romance novels. I love them, absolutely love them, but the only time I have to read them is when I travel. And I sleep best when I travel."

Lawrence adds, "And when you travel you stay in a hotel, which you associate with a good night's rest. So if the only time you read that type of book is as you transition to rest, you will learn to associate that type of book with rest. Kind of like an infant hearing a lullaby before you put her to rest. I sang the same lullaby to by my baby girl every time I would put her to rest. And as a toddler, anytime she would hear that same lullaby, she would yawn.

"Six: Do not go to bed angry. Fair enough. That is good overall life advice. But what about when you are feeling stressed, upset, nervous or anxious? All of these are wake-promoting emotions and thoughts that cause your mind to race. The fear of not sleeping also causes feelings of hope-lessness. It makes you feel like you are a victim of circum-stances out of your control.

"Seven: Do not study or work in bed. This goes both ways. When people study in bed what generally happens? They fall asleep because they associate the bed with sleep. Well like-wise, you don't want to introduce a daytime activity to bed. Other things include conducting important work prior to bed-time, doing bills, organizing your schedule, doing taxes, do-ing laundry, watching TV, reading, studying, snacking, thinking, planning and worrying."

Mellissa interjects, "Funny you say that because I always studied in bed in college. On nights that I had exams, I would study all night in bed. To change positions sometimes I would go to the floor and when I did that I would always end up falling asleep on the floor instead of my bed."

Lawrence nods. "So early in college you started associat-ing your bed with trying to force yourself to be awake. It's just like when someone can't sleep in bed, they get up and go to the couch and end up falling asleep there.

"Eight: Have a comfortable mattress. Again, fair enough. But comfort is variable and it's more important to avoid sleep-ing on a bed that is perceived as uncomfortable. The room is also important. Keep it dark and quiet. You don't want blinds open with streetlights and jackhammers.

"Nine: Use the bed for sleep or sex only. But what if one doesn't enjoy sex? I have had some post-menopausal women tell me they rather do laundry than have sex. It creates a nega-tive connotation about the bed; the mind gets wired if the bed is associated with discomfort.

"Ten: Do not drink caffeine at night. This is a good one. Even mild amounts of caffeine, such as iced tea, have been shown to cause problems with getting to sleep and staying asleep. But it doesn't end there. Substances overall need to be addressed. Nicotine suppresses REM sleep but also keeps you alert."

Mellissa furrows her brows. "So when I can't sleep and I go outside and smoke, it is waking me up more?"

"Physically, yes. But psychologically you also start to worry about your husband catching you.

"We are done. I will send you the bill in six weeks. If you are not sleeping better regularly, you have the right to refuse payment under the condition you call me and tell me why."

Mellissa sits up and starts putting her shoes back on. "That's it? Just tell you why?"

"Yes, Mellissa. It is actually written in the contract. Tell me why."

"Why exactly would you want to know why?" Mellissa straps on her right shoe.

Lawrence takes out his iPad. "Because I'm keeping a list. Just like a business may have a page of frequently asked questions, I'm keeping a list of encountered sleep complaints. These treatments work. And for the life of me, I just don't understand why they are applied only for cases of chronic insomnia. I have only had a few people give me the personal call and the information I was able to get from them was more valuable than the price of the sessions. I have been accumulating some sleep pearls and have called them Paradise Sleep Pearls."

"Nice." Mellissa smiles and nods.

Lawrence returns the smile. "Any other curious questions?"

"Just one. What was your dog's name?"

"Agrypnia! He was a rescue dog and old when I got him. He barked at night so I called him, Agrypnia. One moment I would be counting sheep to sleep, the next moment I can't sleep because of Agrypnia."

Mellissa gets up, picks up her purse and chuckles inside.

They say their goodbyes and just as she closes the door, she hears, "Don't forget to call, but hopefully you won't!"

Paradise Sleep Pearls: Sleep hygiene is indeed important. These are daily living activities that are inconsistent with the maintenance of good sleep. Look around your sleep environment and think LEARNS: Light, Environment, Activity, Routine, Napping, Substances.

Drake, C. Behavioral Sleep Medicine Series: Sleep Hygiene Webinar. American Academy of Sleep Medicine. 2009, May.

Stubborn as a Stick

After Mellissa leaves Paradise Sleep, she doesn't head straight to the airport. She detours back to the hotel. Scurries to the outdoor bar and says, "OK Palo. Its day six. So what's your story?"

"You ask me again so I will tell you." Palo stopped and held a pitcher of ice water for a moment then he proceeds. "I was born to a wealthy family in Naples. What in America you call Old Money."

"Did your family lose the money?" It seemed like a logical question, as he was a bartender now on the other side of the world.

"No. My father actually began to dabble into the fashion industry, later he controlled it. We moved to Paris when I was a boy. Today we are billionaires. You can call us New Money just as well. I do not have enough time in this lifetime to spend all our money?"

"It's not every day you hear that!"

"I told you that you would not believe me." Palo turns his back and puts away the water pitcher.

"Did you do something to upset your family?"

"Our family is very loving. Though, I once upset my family and changed our lives. When I was 20, I took my father's motorcycle. I had been courting a very beautiful bella, like yourself for over a year and finally we were connecting. We had a great night, dancing, dinning. On my way, all I can think about was my bella. I saw a red traffic light, but all I thought about was her red lips. It didn't occur to stop. I crashed into police car and flew off the bike. I almost died. I was in the hospital for a long time.

"At first, when the sedation wore off, all I felt was pain and all I heard was crying. I could hear my mother screaming, *Antonio!* I could hear my bella crying my name as well. I was in a full body cast. I could not move; I could only cry."

"I thought your name was Palo?"

"Let me finish. When I got out of the hospital, I had difficulty sleeping."

Mellissa sat up straight.

"In the hospital, they would always give me medication for pain, they seemed to know when the pain would come and give me pills before it was a problem. At home, however, I started drinking wine instead. My mother would tell me to take the pain medications they gave me. I told my mother, 'No!' I never explained why. My mother told me I was stubborn. That I was as hardheaded as the wooden sticks that they use to drive the Gondola's in Venice, a palo. And that I would rather keep my head under water so I did not have to face reality."

"What did your father say?"

"He told me it was time to make changes in life. My father told me that he believed university education was too often wasted on the young. He wanted me to see the world, but he also said that I also had to learn the value of hard work. So when I got better after the accident, we made a deal that he would send me around the world for three months at a time, but that first I needed to learn the value of hard work for three months at a time. He said minimum one year. After that, he would pay for whatever university I wanted to go to. It sounded like the greatest deal in the world of a young man, fun but fair."

"What about the girl who you took out on the bike?"

"Ah, yes, she said she loved me that night. I knew she was for me and I knew she would marry me one day. She would cry at my bedside every day, at first. My best friend would always be there to pat her on the back. At first, I was so grateful I had such a good friend to help her out. Then she started coming less, crying less and the last time I saw her in the hospital, I pretended my eyes were closed. I opened them just enough when she said goodbye, this time without a kiss to my head. I saw them holding hands on the way out."

"So when did you learn about Paradise Sleep?" Mellissa asks.

"Actually, it is when I accepted that I could not sleep without alcohol and after landing in New York City. My first night there, I could not sleep. So I did what I knew would work, I went into a bar to get a drink. But when I walked in, it was hard to get service. It was so busy. I saw the look of stress on the owner's face from being understaffed. I approached him and said I was new to the city and that I was looking for work. He paused. I told him I was either going to sit in his bar and make it busier than it was already or I was going to be the best bartender he ever had. He looked at me and said, 'You are stubborn, but convincing.' I told him I am stubborn as a stick and my name is Palo. He then gave me an apron and I cleared every table and started mixing drinks."

"But that doesn't answer how you ended up in Florida?"

Palo smiles and leans forward on the bar. "I decided to start reading American literature to pass the time. It was something to make an effort to get my mind off sleep. The first book I picked up was by Earnest Hemmingway. I was fascinated. I decided I wanted to experience his inspiration. So one day I packed my bags and bought a ticket to Key West. On the flight, I was flipping through the magazine. I saw an advertisement for Paradise Sleep.

"Later I found out through Lawrence that my insomnia started in the hospital, it was a traumatic event to begin with. Life threatening, life changing. But also when I looked back, the curtains were closed all day, the TV was on all night. I had my days and nights mixed up. Nurses would wake me up and ask me how I am sleeping. I swear I went crazy. I saw hallucinations. Lawrence explained it to me. I was so sleep deprived that at times I would sleep while I seemed awake. I about lost my mind and was afraid to sleep."

"I'm sorry to hear you went through so much." Mellissa places a hand of comfort on his. "But just the sleep retreat cured your insomnia."

"Don't feel sorry for me because I'm not sorry for myself. But no, the sleep retreat for me was the first step. Lawrence realized that I had trauma, PTSD from the accident. I also had depression from losing my bella; I had to go to counseling for that."

"What about now?"

"I have new dreams of opening the finest restaurant in the world that has a touch of my Italian culture, my French upbringing with a twist of Florida. The citrus, the ocean and Latin influence. My family is proud and supports me. They come and visit. They love this area so much they bought a house on Sanibel."

Mellissa laughed.

"You are going to miss your plane." Palo takes her hands. "You can come back for a mojito anytime with your husband or you can come to my restaurant when I open it. I want to open it in Vegas. I want to prove to myself that I can sleep in the city that never sleeps."

They both laugh and exchange emails. As Mellissa drives towards the airport, she ruminates. *Why does he continue to be around alcohol?*

Paradise Sleep Pearls: Alcohol is commonly self-prescribed to aid in sleep onset. Though the sedative effect may help one get to sleep, the physical effects later in the night include decreased deep sleep, decreased REM sleep and increased night wakening. The sleep disturbance may be from subsequent tachycardia and sweating. Also, alcohol can relax the airway and make an obstructive sleep apnea worse.

1. Roehrs T, Roth T. Sleep, sleepiness and alcohol use. Alcohol Res Health. 2001; 25(2): 101-09.
2. Brower KJ. Alcohol's effects on sleep in alcoholics. Alcohol Res Health. 2001; 25(2): 110-25.

There's No Place Like Home

The entire flight back to Nashville, Mellissa daydreams about her wild experiences. What stands out more than anything are moments of serenity.

She enjoys dinner on the porch with Rick. She shares all she has learned about sleep, the people she met and about her. They clean up and head to bed. Lying and facing each other, Mellissa, in her new pajamas, asks, "How is the CPAP?"

"Wonderful! I told the sleep doctor that I was having problems. He put it into perspective for me. He said none of us were born with a mask on our face. It can take time to adjust. He gave me a sample of a mask liner, a thin cloth to put on the plastic. The leak is gone now."

"So I won't have to nudge you anymore?"

"Nope. No more nudging. But you aren't going to find me sexy anymore when I have the mask on."

"You want a news flash? You're snoring isn't sexy."

"Hey, you are actually wearing pajamas to bed." Rick reaches for her pajama pants, puts his fingers on the silk tie, then pulls it untied.

"I can tell you're excited to see me."

Rick reaches over to Mellissa, takes his finger and tucks some hair behind her ear. He kisses her forehead.

Mellissa smiles.

He kisses the prominence of her cheek.

She giggles as the warmth of his air also tickles.

He then places his lips gently on Mellissa's ear and he whispers, "So the bed is for sleep and *what* only."

Paradise Sleep Pearls: Incidence of OSA (Obstructive Sleep Apnea) in males from 30-60 years of age has been estimated at approximately 25%. To place this in perspective, the incidence of asthma in the general population is about 5%.

Half of patients with OSA may complain of Insomnia. Also, nearly half of patients on chronic hypnotic medications have an undiagnosed/untreated OSA, and potentially the hypnotic medications could be further provoking OSA by pharyngeal muscle relaxation.

1. Young T et al. The occurrence of sleep-disordered breathing among middle-aged adults. N Engl J Med 1993; 328
2. Krell SB, Kapur VK. Sleep Breathing. 2005; 9:104-10
3. Smith S, et al. Sleep Med. 2004; 5:449-456

Positive Vibes

"Sleep is the new sex, everybody wants it and Paradise Sleep is the Sandman," Mellissa tells her sister Dedee while they are out to lunch. More than a month has gone by since Mellissa's sleep retreat and she has stuck with the sleep diet. Mellissa works long hours during the week and her sister has been busy with her two kids, so this is the first time they've been able to catch up.

"So I guess it was good for you?" Dedee asks.

"It was unique."

"Why? Did they brainwash you?"

"No. You'll never believe what happened while I was there."

"Well, what did you learn? Did they put you on melatonin?"

How do I explain days of sessions and processing information over a lunch? Mellissa decides to summarize everything. "You feel the way that you think."

"OK...what does that have to do with sleep?"

"I don't know how to explain it." Mellissa twists her head and looks up at the clouds thoughtfully.

"Try me! If I get bored, I'll start talking about my kids. If I like what I hear, I'll send them there. Lately, I have to rock the baby to sleep in my arms, and the older one, I can't get to sleep through the night unless it's in our bed."

"That's a good start, actually. You know, many times when I was up at night, I would obsess about getting pregnant. I would tell myself that if I didn't get pregnant, Rick would leave me."

"That's absurd! You guys are so awesome together. You're soul mates. Besides, there are so many other options. You could adopt or even do in vitro. Why would you think that?"

"I had a relationship that ended in an argument once. I guess everyone has. When I don't sleep, well I'm pretty cranky the next day. I can be short tempered and you always worry that one bad fight can ruin a relationship. Well, I would think about my infertility and about being cranky and fighting. I believed that if I didn't get pregnant he would leave me." Mellissa feels the vibration of a text, but she silences her phone without looking at the screen. "Just the thought of a fight leading to the end of a relationship makes me feel bad." Mellissa gets another text alert, the phone vibrates and she pushes it to the side.

Dessert comes, signaling their lunch date is almost over. Mellissa no longer wants to indulge in deep thought or conversation. She wants to laugh and enjoy the rest of their time together.

"You know what else I learned? Psychologists are not psychiatrists and they are not psychics, either. Florida state troopers don't have balls and some dogs have no tails!"

Mellissa's sister laughs but looks confused.

Mellissa recaps her unexpected twists and turns through Sanibel and Southwest Florida. Her encounters with Sam, Lawrence and Cindy all entertain her sister. The tangled intertwining of people's lives leaves her sister dumbfounded. The stories seem to satisfy her sister's need for gossip.

"Wow! What a trip," Dedee exclaims. "What did Jez think of your trip?"

"Jez signed up. She's working just during the day now, but she keeps snoozing her alarm each morning and has been showing up late to work. Her manager is becoming increasingly impatient with her. Jez wants to find out why she functions better at night."

"Wow. Maybe she has a misaligned body clock?" Dedee then curiously eyes Mellissa. "Mellissa, you haven't gone outside for a cigarette. Did they tell you how to quit smoking as well?"

"No. I just realized on the trip that I don't *need* nicotine. What I need is to set time aside and take deep calming exhalations."

"I don't understand? Isn't nicotine addictive?"

"Setting aside time to relax is addictive. Deep exhalations have always relaxed me. Remember when we were kids and we would drink warm milk prior to going to bed?"

"Yes. I never understood why you liked it so hot that you would then have to blow on it." Dedee's eyes grow wide and she smiles. "You mean blowing on the steam is what relaxes you?"

"I figured I don't fall asleep if I put milk or creamer in my coffee. Deep, slow exhalations relax me. Blowing the steam from the milk was like smoking to blow off some steam. That's my theory on why I hadn't been successful in smoking cessation before. I never crave nicotine replacements. I look back and realize that the slower and longer I would exhale the smoke, the more relaxed I felt. Before now, I hadn't replaced the time I set to myself to evoke a relaxation response."

Mellissa gets a third text. "It's probably Rick," she says, pulling out her phone. "Yeah, it's him and he sent a picture." Mellissa looks at the phone and waits for the picture to download.

Mellissa looks back to her phone. Her eyes widen as her mouth drops open.

"Mel, you have me worried. What is it?"

Mellissa can't speak. Her eyes tear and from her ears to neck, she is bright red. She suddenly laughs and cries at the same time.

"What is it, Mellissa?"

Mellissa hands the phone over to her sister. She can see the + sign on the pregnancy test in the picture.

"Your husband is pregnant?" she asks, half-seriously.

"No, out of habit I take a pregnancy test once a month since my period is so irregular. I never expect them to come back positive so sometimes while I have to wait for the results, I do other things and forget to go back and check the test."

"I'm so happy for you, Mel! You are going to be a great mom and Rick is going to love shopping with you, and daddy's little girl."

"We'll see! He says he only makes boys."

The girls laugh and cry. They eventually wear out their welcome at the restaurant.

Paradise Sleep Pearls: The grand theory of why people sleep remains a mystery. It obviously has a function given its complexity. Functions of sleep are vast. Restorative and growth functions include release of growth hormone during deep sleep. Metabolic regulations that occur include energy conservation and removal of toxins generated during wakefulness. Neuronal growth, brain development and restoration, and learning and memory consolidation all occur during sleep.

Shwartz, D. Neurobiology and Function of Sleep. 12th Annual Current Concepts in Sleep. 2010, September. Tampa, FL

Afterword

This labor of love is not about any one single patient. The stories told here are amalgams of stories I have come across through clinical care, conferences, webinars, readings, and in some cases, personal experience (the insomnia experience).

Lawrence is fictional and is not me. Lawrence was made to be more entertaining than practical and is no more of a real therapist then Ken Jeong is in Couples Retreat.

There are several effective treatments for insomnia including meditation, yoga, clinical hypnosis and biofeedback to name a few. Each of these approaches centers our attention and stimulates a relaxation response, such as described by Harvard doctor Herbert Benson, M.D. in his ground breaking book *The Relaxation Response*.

Mindfulness and self-hypnosis have been effective for me in combination with the discussions of the behavioral sleep medicine topics in the five sessions. In this story, it seems as if Mellissa almost picked up on meditation without extensive coaching. Part of the reason is I have found that "reading" about meditation was not an effective way for me to learn. That may not be true for everyone. However, for me I began to learn about meditation when I experienced it, verbally, with someone guiding the meditation.

This book was meant as a creative way to raise awareness of insomnia. Other sleep disorders such as circadian rhythm sleep disorders, behavioral insomnia of childhood, lucid dreaming, caretaker insomnia, sleep eating disorders and other parasomnias are all different stories for a different day. For the purposes of fiction, several steps of an appropriate sleep evaluation were skipped. If you suffer from insomnia or excessive daytime sleepiness, several steps should be taken prior to engaging in any type of behavioral or medicinal therapy, including self-medication with herbals or over-the-counter sleep aids.

The primary care physician should conduct a medical evaluation to ensure there are no underlying medical conditions causing the symptoms. The primary care physician should also screen for psychological disorders—with caution, since sleep disorders can have psychological symptoms as well. I also advise that a board-certified sleep physician also conduct a history and physical because there are many sleep disorders that can cause symptoms of fatigue, sleepiness and even insomnia.

What I most hope to create is a ripple effect. I want people to go back to their doctors and encourage them to learn about behavioral sleep medicine. I want doctors to go back to their medical schools and ask, "Why didn't you teach us about sleep?" I want practicing psychologists to challenge themselves to learn more about sleep.

"When you plant a seed you need to water it. The rose isn't going to just bloom."

—*Mariann Suarez, Ph.D.* on Motivational Interviewing

Paradise Sleep Pearls: Story and Metaphor.

As I read goodnight stories to my own children, I find myself wondering if the stories take their own imagination when their little eyes rest. I also wonder at what point they understand the metaphors. Is it before the lights are turned off or the next day when they're approached with real life situations and they have learned not to cry wolf or that slow and steady wins the race?

The Sleep Diet teaches sleep science through story. Stories amuse, whereas facts illuminate. Embedded within this story are also metaphors. Some are direct, whereas others are permissive.

I believe in living life in the present moment, metaphorically I wrote the story in the present tense. Each character has traits that represent a broad spectrum of everyday real life situations. I wonder what you allowed the characters to mean to you.

When reading this story, some may have initial consuming thoughts of character names, coincidences or stereotypes. And through the journey of the story, they may have allowed themselves to dismiss the thoughts and learn the intended sleep science. All who have read through this book have shown motivation in their journey of achieving better sleep (or helping others achieve better sleep).

Allow yourself each night to use your imagination towards images of what paradise is to you, in a way that provides a portal of escape from your daily stresses. Or perhaps you may want to imagine your own version of what happened to the characters and what they mean to you. When you awaken from your restful and peaceful sleep, I invite you to share your stories and metaphors on www.ParadiseSleep.com.

1. Pink DH. A Whole New Mind, Why Right-Brainers Will Rule The Future. Riverhead Books. New York. 2005
2. Hammond DC. Handbook of Hypnotic Suggestions and Metaphors. W. W. Norton and Company, Inc. New York. 1990

Acknowledgments

To my beautiful wife, Krystal, the contents of this book have indeed divided my time, but not my love for you. Thank you for your support and understanding.

When I think of beauty, I think of her.
When I look at my children, I thank God they look like her.
When I close my eyes, I see her.
When I think of love, I envision her.
She is on my mind night and day.
She is in my thoughts in every way.
I can't express with words how much I love her.
But I'll never stop trying.

To my children Manuel and Jada, you inspire me in ways words cannot explain. You were my inspiration to start Paradise Sleep. You kids drive my desire to make this world a better place. Daddy loves you.

To my parents, friends, and loved ones, thank you for your faith and encouragement through every step in life. Always tell people you love that you love them, and always be true to yourself. Go Bucs!

So many people helped me in the process of writing this book. One thing I have learned is the term, "It's a man's world" is a giant façade. Anytime I have needed help in life, and in particular with this book, women have provided the best help. Women are the backbone of our society.

Paradise Sleep Pearls: Smiling makes you feel good. The nerves of our muscles of facial expression come from our brainstem. The brainstem also has connections to our limbic system, which is our emotional area. The brainstem has other nerves that communicate with the emotional limbic area that then go back to our body, including our heart and other organs in our body. In feelings of happiness, we are contracting muscles that raise the cheek in combination, which pulls up the corners of the lips. This also sends input to our emotional area and to our body as well as it gives a "heartfelt" feeling.

Tell a child you love their smile. When you compliment their smile, they will grow confidence in their smile. When they smile more, they will feel better and their self-esteem will grow.

1. Gladwell M. Blink. The Power of Thinking Without Even Thinking. 2005. Back Bay Books. New York
2. Bradberry, T. and Greaves, J. Emotional Intelligence 2.0 2009. TalentSmart. San Diego, CA

Testimonials

"Dr. Colon has written an ingenious book that teaches you how to improve your sleep. This book uses the vehicle of an engaging and hilarious novel to share essential wisdom about sleep disorders and how to improve sleep. You will not want to put it down and you will learn exactly how to sleep better as you enjoy the story about a woman's journey to solve her sleep issues. If you ever have trouble sleeping or suffer with any type of sleep disorder this book will help you sleep better tonight!"

Debra Burdick, LCSWR, BCN, author of *Mindfulness Skills Workbook for Clinicians and Clients* and *ADHD and Sleep.*

"As a female executive trying to balance the rigors of work, family, social life, and general well being, *The Sleep Diet* aids in creating a road map to a healthy and full life. A unique and inspiring read that uses a fictional story to help the reader connect to the deeper issues and realities of sleep disorders, Dr. Jose Colon explores the mentality of the sleep deprived with unexpected twists and turns all the way through to the end. The end of each chapter delivers fantastic guidance and invaluable information that can lead to some much needed shut eye."

Rachel Bookbinder, Vice President of Nirvana Mattress

"*The Sleep Diet*, a spellbinding short novel that will keep you laughing, musing, and turning the page to learn more about how the field of behavioral sleep medicine can help you start sleeping better tonight. *The Sleep Diet* offers natural and easy solutions for anyone, insomniac or not, who is looking for a healthy night's rest."

Dr. Susanne K. Long, Ph.D. of Psychological and Life Skills Associates, licensed clinical psychologist and nationally certified school psychologist

"*The Sleep Diet* is a book I highly recommend for anyone who has ever had sleep issues or who is just looking for a great read. This novel is not only entertaining, but it covers a variety of subjects that the majority of men and women can relate to. Dr. Jose Colon is brilliant in making this novel compelling and incredibly easy to read, while educating readers at the same time. It is rare to find an entertaining book that can teach you along the way."

Dr. Magdalena Battles, Ph.D., Board of Directors for Miracles in Action and a life coach with affiliation to the American Psychological Association and American Counseling Association

"Dr. Colon's approach to sleep education and to the treatment of sleep disorders– specifically insomnia in this offering– is unique, and frankly, a lot of fun. In his book *The Sleep Diet* he introduces us to the main character who struggles to understand her sleep disorder and how it impacts every aspect of her life. This book is not your typical self-help book. Instead, Dr. Colon provides us with an engaging and funny case-based learning experience. We aren't simply told the facts, as in a text book, then provided lists of instructions to follow. We are placed right in the middle of Mellissa's sleep-less life as she tries to understand and ultimately overcome her disorder."

Patricia Ritch MD, PhD., member of the American Academy of Sleep Medicine, Diplomate, American Board of Psychiatry and Neurology, Diplomate, Baylor Scott & White Healthcare

About the Author

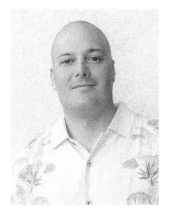

Dr. Jose Colon is the founder of *Paradise Sleep*, Inc.™, an organization dedicated to education of sleep health topics that impact public health. Dr. Colon is dual board certified in sleep medicine and neurology with special qualifications in child neurology. He has Masters in Public Health in Child and Maternal Health. He is a founding member of the Society of Behavioral Sleep Medicine and a member of the American Society of Clinical Hypnosis. Dr. Colon resides in Southwest Florida with his wife and two young children. He encourages all families that a healthy child needs a healthy family.

CPSIA information can be obtained
at www.ICGtesting.com
Printed in the USA
LVHW081236141218
600306LV00005B/10/P